The ESSE of

Microbiology

Tammy S. Race McCormick, M.S.

Former Instructor
Department of Biological Sciences
Northern Kentucky University
Highland Heights, KY

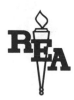 *Research & Education Association*
61 Ethel Road West
Piscataway, New Jersey 08854

THE ESSENTIALS®
OF MICROBIOLOGY

Year 2004 Printing

Printed in the United States of America

Library of Congress Control Number 00-134283

International Standard Book Number 0-87891-924-4

WHAT "THE ESSENTIALS" WILL DO FOR YOU

This book is a review and study guide. It is comprehensive and it is concise.

It helps in preparing for exams and in doing homework, and remains a handy reference source at all times.

It condenses the vast amount of detail characteristic of the subject matter and summarizes the **essentials** of the field.

It will thus save hours of study and preparation time.

The book provides quick access to the important facts, principles, concepts, practices, and definitions in the field.

Materials needed for exams can be reviewed in summary form— eliminating the need to read and re-read many pages of textbook and class notes. The summaries will even tend to bring detail to mind that had been previously read or noted.

This "ESSENTIALS" book has been prepared by experts in the field, and has been carefully reviewed to ensure accuracy and maximum usefulness.

Dr. Max Fogiel
Program Director

ACKNOWLEDGMENTS

We would like to thank Angela H. Kaya, Ph.D., Cindy Coe Taylor, Ph.D., and Jay M. Templin, Ed.D., for their editorial contributions.

CONTENTS

Chapter No.		Page No.

1 HISTORY AND SCOPE OF MICROBIOLOGY   1
1.1 Early History 1
1.2 The Golden Age of Microbiology 2
1.3 Later Discoveries and the Beginnings of Virology 4
1.4 Scope of Microbiology 4

2 EQUIPMENT AND TECHNIQUES   5
2.1 Units of Measurement 5
2.2 Microscopes 5
2.3 Preparation of Specimens for Light Microscopy 9
2.4 Staining 10
2.5 Culturing Microorganisms 12

3 SURVEY OF MICROORGANISMS   17
3.1 Prokaryotes and Eukaryotes 17
3.2 Bacteria 19
3.3 The Eukaryotic Cell 26
3.4 Viruses 34

4 MICROBIAL METABOLISM   38
4.1 General Terms 38
4.2 Enzymes 38
4.3 Oxidation and Reduction 39
4.4 Phosphorylation 40
4.5 Carbohydrate Catabolism 40
4.6 Lipid and Protein Catabolism 43
4.7 Photosynthesis 43
4.8 Other Anabolic Pathways 44

| 4.9 | Nutritional Modes | 44 |

5	**TRANSPORT OF MOLECULES**	**46**
5.1	Transport	46
5.2	Simple Diffusion	46
5.3	Osmosis	46
5.4	Facilitated Diffusion	47
5.5	Active Transport	47
5.6	Group Translocation	47
5.7	Endocytosis and Exocytosis	48

6	**BACTERIAL GROWTH**	**49**
6.1	Growth of Bacterial Populations	49
6.2	Ways to Measure Growth of Bacterial Populations	51
6.3	Physical and Chemical Requirements for Growth	52

7	**CONTROL OF MICROBIAL GROWTH— DISINFECTION AND ANTISEPSIS**	**55**
7.1	General Terms	55
7.2	Factors Influencing Disinfectant Activity	56
7.3	Physical Methods	56
7.4	Chemical Disinfection and Sterilization	58
7.5	Evaluating a Disinfectant	58
7.6	Microbial Death	60

8	**CONTROL OF MICROBIAL GROWTH— ANTIMICROBIAL CHEMOTHERAPY**	**61**
8.1	General Terms	61
8.2	Types of Agents	62
8.3	Mechanisms of Action of Antimicrobial Drugs	63
8.4	Evaluating an Antimicrobial Drug	65
8.5	Side Effects	65
8.6	Drug Resistance	65
8.7	Some Common Antibacterial Drugs	66

9	**MICROBIAL GENETICS**	**68**
9.1	Genetics	68
9.2	Chromosomes	68
9.3	Replication	70
9.4	Transcription–Synthesis of RNA	70
9.5	Translation	71
9.6	Mutation	72
9.7	Gene Transfer	74
9.8	Recombination	76
9.9	Transposons	76
9.10	Recombinant DNA Technology	76
9.11	Diversity and Evolution	78
9.12	Regulation of Gene Expression in Bacteria	78
10	**ROLES OF MICROBES IN DISEASE**	**80**
10.1	Host–Microbe Relationships	80
10.2	Kinds of Disease	81
10.3	How Microbes Cause Disease	82
10.4	The Disease Process	85
10.5	Koch's Postulates	85
10.6	Epidemiology	86
10.7	Host Defense Mechanisms	88
10.8	Microbial Diseases of the Skin and Eyes	95
10.9	Microbial Diseases of the Respiratory System	96
10.10	Microbial Diseases of the Digestive System	96
10.11	Microbial Diseases of the Cardiovascular System	97
10.12	Microbial Diseases of the Nervous System	98
10.13	Microbial Diseases of the Genitourinary System	98
11	**MICROBES IN THE ENVIRONMENT**	**100**
11.1	Microbes and the Recycling of Nutrients	100
11.2	Bioremediation	101

12   MICROBES IN INDUSTRY   102

12.1   Microbes in the Food Industry 102

12.2   Industrial Microbiology 102

12.3   Microbes and Medicine 103

12.4   Microbes and Recombinant DNA Technology 103

CHAPTER 1

History and Scope of Microbiology

1.1 Early History

Microbiology is the study of microbes (microorganisms), i.e., organisms too small to be observed by the naked eye, and dates back to the seventeenth century, when Hans and Zaccharias **Janssen** (ca. 1600) invented the first compound microscope.

Robert **Hooke** (1665) made early observations using a compound microscope. From his observations of cork, he coined the word "cell" to describe the "little boxes" he saw as the smallest structures of life, setting the foundation for "cell theory."

The **cell theory** states that all living things are composed of cells.

Anton **van Leeuwenhoek** (1670s and 1680s) was first to observe and describe living microbes, which he referred to as "animalcules." His homemade microscopes magnified specimens up to 200x–300x.

Carolus **Linnaeus** (1735) developed a general system of classification and **binomial nomenclature** (genus name + specific epithet or species name).

The theory of **spontaneous generation**—which states that new life can arise from nonliving matter—was commonly accepted until the mid-1880s.

Francesco **Redi** (1660s) was first to present experimental evidence to refute spontaneous generation. Redi used cloth-covered jars to show that maggots do not arise spontaneously in meat but that the meat must be open to contact with flies in order for maggots to appear. However, his results were not accepted by many (the experiment that finally put the theory of spontaneous generation to rest did not occur for another 200 years!—see **Pasteur**, section 1.2).

John **Needham** (1740s) published experimental evidence in support of spontaneous generation. In his experiments, he showed that nutrient solutions could be boiled, and yet when cooled, microorganisms would soon appear. In the 1760s, Lazzaro **Spallanzani** countered this with experiments demonstrating that if such flasks were sealed, the microorganisms did not appear after boiling. **Needham** and his supporters argued that the boiling was responsible for killing some "vital force" (later thought to be oxygen upon its discovery) and that sealing the flask prevented its re-entry. It was still another hundred years before Pasteur's experiments disproved the theory.

On the medical front, Edward **Jenner** (1798) developed and tested the first **vaccine**. Jenner noticed that milkmaids exposed to cowpox rarely developed the more serious smallpox. He then used cowpox to successfully inoculate patients against smallpox.

Ignaz Philipp **Semmelweis** (1840s) noticed a connection between doctors doing autopsies and patients developing **puerperal (childbirth) fever**; he was first to suggest that doctors should wash their hands between procedures.

1.2   The Golden Age of Microbiology

The **Golden Age of Microbiology** (1850-1890) was a period during which major historical figures established microbiology as a viable scientific discipline.

Louis **Pasteur**—disproof of spontaneous generation/proof of biogenesis (1861). Pasteur devised a special kind of flask (the **swan necked flask**) in order to disprove spontaneous generation. Swan neck flasks are not sealed off; rather, the neck of the flask is open, but is long and curved. Such flasks are open to air and to any "vital force." However, microorganisms from the outer air become trapped in the curved neck of the flask and are thus prevented from contaminating the medium. Infusions or nutrient broths that have been sterilized by boiling do not become contaminated in such a flask unless the neck becomes broken. Thus, Pasteur disproved spontaneous generation while demonstrating that the inoculating (contaminating) organisms are present in the air.

Pasteur was first to show that microorganisms are *everywhere*, including the air. This discovery provided impetus for the development of **aseptic techniques** in the laboratory and medical situations to prevent contamination.

Pasteur was also instrumental in work on the role of yeast and other microorganisms in **fermentation** or the conversion of sugars to alcohol. He developed a heating process used to kill bacteria in some alcoholic beverages and milk, i.e., **pasteurization**.

Pasteur was also a pioneer in the area of immunology. He developed "vaccines" (he coined the term) for chicken cholera and rabies (1884). In his search for a rabies vaccine, Pasteur used the brain tissue of rabid animals to inoculate rabbits. He then used the dried spinal cords of those rabbits to inoculate experimental animals. In 1865, he used this treatment to successfully vaccinate a young boy who had been bitten by a rabid dog, and showing signs of the disease, was expected to die. The vaccine worked and the boy lived. (Modern **vaccines** are generally live, avirulent microorganisms, or killed pathogens or components isolated from pathogens, especially by use of recombinant DNA techniques.)

It was one of Pasteur's publications (1857) that laid the foundation for the **germ theory of disease** by suggesting that microorganisms are the *cause* of disease rather than the *result* of it. This theory states that microorganisms can invade other organisms and are responsible for the transmission of infectious diseases.

Joseph **Lister** (1860s) introduced the use of disinfectants to clean surgical dressings and instruments. Robert **Koch's** work (1870s) provided further support for the germ theory of disease. His work with the sheep disease **anthrax** was instrumental in establishing the concept of "one disease—one organism," which is the foundation of medical microbiology. He was the first to establish **pure culture technique**, and the first to use agar in growth medium. **Koch's postulates** (1876; see section 10.5) are still used today as the appropriate method for demonstrating that a specific microorganism transmits a specific disease.

1.3   Later Discoveries and the Beginnings of Virology

Virology had its beginnings in 1892 when Dmitri **Ivanowski** showed that the organism responsible for tobacco mosaic disease was able to pass through filters that stopped all known bacteria. Wendell **Stanley** (1935) later demonstrated that this organism was fundamentally different from other known organisms and could even be crystallized. The development of the electron microscope in the 1940s paved the way for further understanding and study of viruses.

Paul **Ehrlich** (1910) was first to use chemicals to treat disease (chemotherapy). His search for a "magic bullet" that would kill the cells of the infecting microorganism but not those of the host led to the discovery of Salvarsan in 1910. This chemotherapeutic agent was used in the treatment of syphilis. Along with Ehrlich's work, the discoveries of penicillin in 1928 by Alexander **Fleming** and sulfa drugs in 1932 by Gerhard **Domagk** ushered in our modern era of chemotherapy.

1.4   Scope of Microbiology

Microorganisms are found in all five kingdoms: Monera, Protista, Fungi, Plantae, and Animalia. All of the Monera (bacteria and cyanophytes) are microorganisms.

There are many fields of microbiology. Study of the classification of microorganisms constitutes **microbial taxonomy**. **Bacteriology** is the study of bacteria; **phycology**, the study of algae; **mycology**, the study of fungi; **protozoology**, the study of protozoans; **parasitology**, the study of parasitic microbes; and **virology**, the study of viruses.

Epidemiology is the study of the distribution and frequency of disease. **Etiology** is the study of the causes of disease. **Immunology** is the study of host defense against disease.

Various fields of **applied microbiology** include food technology, industrial microbiology, medical/pharmaceutical microbiology, genetic engineering, and environmental microbiology.

Microbial metabolism, **microbial genetics**, and **microbial ecology** are all fields of microbiology as well.

CHAPTER 2

Equipment and Techniques

2.1 Units of Measurement

The basic unit of measure is the **meter (1 m = 3.28 ft)**. There are 1,000 millimeters (mm) per meter.

Microbes are generally measured in micrometers (μm) or nanometers (nm).

$$1 \ \mu\text{m} = 0.000001 = 10^{-6} \ \text{m}$$
$$1 \ \text{nm} = 10^{-9} \ \text{m}$$

2.2 Microscopes

Microscopy is the process of projecting energy (visible light, ultraviolet light, or electrons) onto an object, and then using the energy that is emitted from that object to create an image on a sensing device (e.g., the lens of your eye, a screen, or a photographic film). Microscopes may differ in the kind of energy used, type of sensing device, resolution, wavelength, and magnification.

Resolution refers to the ability to distinguish adjacent objects or structures as separate and discrete entities. The **resolving power** of a microscope indicates the size of the smallest objects that can be clearly observed.

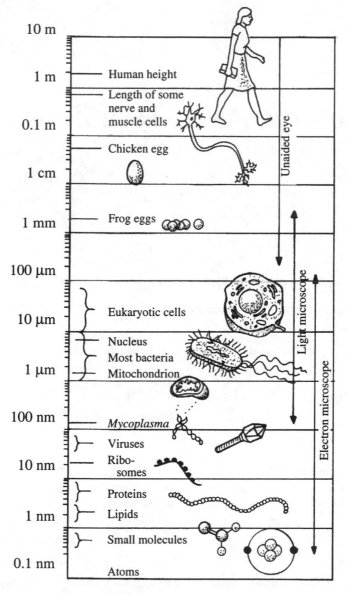

Figure 2.1 Relative Sizes

The limiting factors in resolution are the **wavelength** (λ) of the energy source (e.g., the length of light rays) and the numerical aperture (N.A.) of the lenses.

$$\text{resolving power} = \frac{\lambda}{2 \text{ N.A.}}$$

A **compound light microscope** uses a two-lens system—an ocular lens and an objective lens. Total **magnification** (magnifying power) equals the magnification of the ocular lens *multiplied by* that of the objective lens.

In **bright-field microscopy,** the light is transmitted directly through the specimen. Organisms must generally be stained.

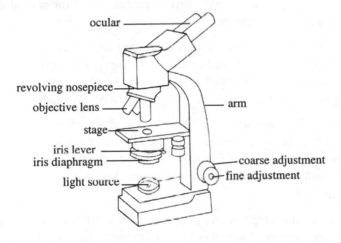

Figure 2.2 The Compound Microscope

Dark-field microscopes have a condenser that reflects light off the specimen at diverse angles and prevents most light from passing directly through the specimen. At the apex of the illuminating cone, light rays are scattered from the specimen into the objective lens and the image is that of a light organism against a dark background. This type of microscope is good for visualizing capsules and in diagnosing diseases caused by spiral bacteria. Even though these organisms are near the limit of resolution, their characteristic movement is discernible in dark-field.

The **phase-contrast** microscope is preferred for the observation of living, unstained organisms. A condenser splits the light beam, throwing the light rays slightly out of phase. Small differences in the densities and refractive indexes of various structures are accentuated, and internal details of live, unstained cells can be observed.

Nomarski (differential interference contrast) microscopes are much like phase-contrast, but the depth of field is very short, resulting in much greater resolution. Images appear to be nearly three-dimensional.

In **fluorescence microscopy,** ultraviolet light is used to excite electrons in molecules. When these electrons fall back to their original energy state, they fluoresce (emit light). Some organisms are naturally fluorescent, but most organisms observed in this way must first be treated with a fluorescent dye or **fluorochrome** (e.g., fluorescein).

A special technique known as **fluorescent antibody staining** or **immunofluorescence** is sometimes used to diagnose an unknown organism. In this case, the fluorochrome is attached to an antibody. Fluorescence indicates that the corresponding antigen is present, thus yielding a positive identification.

Electron microscopes use energy in the form of a beam of electrons rather than a beam of light, and the beam is focused using electromagnets rather than lenses. There are two types of electron microscopes: the transmission electron microscope and the scanning electron microscope. Viruses can be seen only by using electron microscopes.

In **transmission electron microscopy (TEM)**, electrons pass through the specimen. Consequently, TEM cannot be used to view whole organisms; rather, very thin slices (ultrathin sections, e.g., 0.07 μm) are used. TEM sections are generally coated with a heavy metal. TEM is very good for looking at internal structures, and can resolve objects as close as 1 nm, and magnify up to 100,000 times. By using additional photographic enlargement, a total magnification of up to 20 million times may be achieved.

Scanning electron microscopy (SEM) is used to create three-dimensional images of surfaces, both external (whole organism) and internal (via freeze-fracture techniques—see below). SEM specimens are usually coated with an Au/Pd (gold/palladium) alloy or carbon. A magnification of up to 10,000 times, with a resolution of 20 nm, can be achieved (prior to further photographic enlargement). In SEM, electrons are released from the surface of the specimen rather than passing through it. Thus, SEM can provide topographical views of the surfaces of objects in their natural state (without sectioning).

Freeze-fracturing refers to a process wherein a cell is frozen and then cleaved with a knife. This technique can be used with either TEM or SEM to view surfaces or internal structures.

Freeze-etching is a further modification wherein water is evaporated from a freeze-fractured specimen to expose additional surfaces.

Table 2.1 Comparison of Microscopes

	Type of energy	Wavelength	Resolution	Maximum magnification
Light microscope	Visible light	400–700 nm	220 nm	usually 100×, (1,000×–2,000× with oil immersion)
Fluorescence microscope	Ultraviolet light	100–400 nm	110 nm	as above
Electron microscope	Electrons	0.005 nm	1 nm (TEM) 20 nm (SEM)	100,000× (TEM) 10,000× (SEM) prior to photographic enlargement

2.3 Preparation of Specimens for Light Microscopy

Wet mount—a drop of medium containing the organisms is placed on a microscope slide. This technique is used to view living organisms. Carboxymethyl cellulose (2%) can be added to the drop to slow the movement of fast-moving microorganisms.

Hanging drop—a drop is placed on a cover slip that is then inverted over a depression slide. This technique is sometimes used for dark-field illumination.

Smear—used to view dead organisms (the organisms are killed by the process). Microorganisms from a drop of medium are spread across the surface of a glass slide. This smear is air-dried and then heat-fixed (by passing through flame). **Heat fixation** accomplishes three things: (1) it kills the organisms, (2) it causes the organisms to adhere to the slide, and (3) it alters the organisms so that they more readily take up stains.

2.4   Staining

Stain (dye)—a molecule that can bind to a cellular structure and give it color, distinguishing it from the background. In addition to discerning parts of the cell, staining helps to categorize microorganisms, and is used to examine structural and chemical differences in their cell walls. Stains are used extensively in bacterial identification and classification.

Basic (cationic) dyes—positively charged dyes. Examples include methylene blue, crystal violet, safranin, and malachite green. Most bacteria have negatively charged surfaces to which these positively charged dyes are attracted.

Acidic (anionic) dyes—negatively charged dyes (e.g., eosin, picric acid, nigrosin, Congo red). These dyes are often used in **negative staining** wherein the background is stained rather than the organism. With this technique, the cells appear clear against a colored background. It is often used to view capsules. Negative staining avoids heat fixation and chemical reactions; thus, cells appear more natural and less distorted.

Stains may be either **simple** or **differential**.

Simple stain—a single dye is used. It reveals basic cell shapes and arrangements. Examples include methylene blue, safranin, carbolfuchsin, and gentian violet.

Differential stain—two or more dyes are used to distinguish between two kinds of organisms or between two different parts of the same organism. Examples include the Gram stain, Schaeffer-Fulton spore stain, and Ziehl-Neelsen acid-fast stain.

The Gram stain (Christian Gram, 1884)—reveals fundamental differences in the nature of the cell wall (probably due to differences in the amount of peptidoglycan in the cell wall—gram-positive bacteria have more peptidoglycan than do similar gram-negative ones). Often used in bacterial taxonomy, the Gram stain is used on air-dried, heat-fixed (therefore killed) specimens.

2.4.1 The Gram Stain Procedure

The Gram stain procedure includes the following steps (in order):

1. Cells are stained with crystal violet followed by iodine—*all* cells appear purple.

2. Cells are washed with alcohol/acetone—gram-positive organisms remain purple, gram-negative organisms are now clear.

3. Safranin is added to the cells—gram-positive organisms remain purple, gram-negative organisms now appear pink or orange-red.

2.4.2 Mordant

A **mordant,** often an iodine solution, may be added to a staining solution to intensify the stain. The mordant increases the stain's affinity for the specimen or coats the specimen to increase its size and staining ability.

2.4.3 Special Stains

Staining techniques may be specialized for the staining of the capsule, endospores, and flagella.

The **capsule** is a gelatinous coat and is often used as an indicator of virulence. The capsule is water soluble and therefore is removed in normal staining procedures. The capsule is visualized by a staining technique called **negative staining,** in which the specimen is first stained with India ink or nigrosin, which provides a dark background for contrast. The first stain is followed by a simple stain, which appears as a light region around each individual organism.

Endospores are dormant structures that are stained by malachite green and a heating technique to allow the dye to penetrate the cell and the endospores. The endospores are specifically stained by this procedure. Again, to add contrast, a second simple stain usually is added. Thus, endospores appear green within the cellular red/pink background.

Flagella are whiplike structures used in locomotion that require specialized staining methods to increase their thickness. A mordant such as tannic acid or potassium alum is used for this purpose followed by the stain pararosaniline (Leifon method) or carbolfuchsin (Gray method).

2.5 Culturing Microorganisms

A **culture** is a population of microbes living in a culture medium.

Aseptic technique—the prevention of microbial contamination—is critical to pure culture of microorganisms.

2.5.1 Culture Media

A liquid or solid prepared for the purpose of growing microbes is called a nutrient broth or nutrient agar or **culture medium.** A culture medium generally provides the organisms with everything required for their growth, including a carbon source, a nitrogen source, and essential trace elements. Agar, a seaweed derivative, can be used to solidify the medium, which is then called nutrient agar.

A culture medium may be **defined**—in which known quantities of specific nutrients are used and the exact chemical composition is known, or **complex**—in which nutrients of reasonably well-known composition are used, but the exact composition varies from batch to batch, and thus, the exact chemical composition is not known. Synthetic media are chemically defined; natural media are usually complex.

Selective media encourage the growth of some organisms while discouraging the growth of others. Salts, dyes, and antibiotics are among the substances used to inhibit growth of unwanted organisms. An example is mannitol salt agar, which encourages the growth of staphylococci while inhibiting the growth of most other bacteria.

A **differential medium** is one that distinguishes growing microbes on the basis of visible chemical changes in the medium. Reagents in the medium allow for a specific chemical reaction to take place, but only in the presence of particular microorganisms. For example, MacConkey agar contains lactose and red dye; bacteria that can ferment the lactose take up the dye, resulting in the formation of red colonies. Bacteria that cannot ferment lactose form colorless colonies.

A medium can be both differential and selective.

Enrichment medium contains a nutrient (or nutrients) that enhances the growth of particular microbes, e.g., addition of blood to nutrient medium enhances growth of streptococci. This technique is designed to increase the relative numbers of a particular organism; it is possible to obtain pure cultures with this culture method.

Selective media, differential media, and enrichment media are all **diagnostic** media.

Reducing medium is used for the growth of anaerobic organisms. This type of medium contains reducing agents such as thioglycollate or cysteine that will deplete the oxygen levels in the medium.

Liquid medium is used in tightly capped test tubes and heated before use.

Solid medium must be contained in specialized, oxygen-free vessels such as **anaerobic glove boxes** or **anaerobic chambers** such as a GasPak Jar, which uses hydrogen and a palladium catalyst to remove O_2 through the formation of water. Oxygen may also be removed using a vacuum pump and flushing out residual O_2 with nitrogen gas.

2.5.2 Plate Methods

The **streak plate** and the **pour plate** are two techniques for obtaining pure cultures. In both cases, it is assumed that a single bacterial colony arises from a single cell. The number of cells is diluted by the medium in the pour plate method; in the streak plate technique, the number of cells is decreased manually by spreading the inoculum over the surface of the agar medium.

Inoculating loops are sterilized by passing them directly through a flame, to the point of redness. **Flaming** is also used to sterilize the tips of test tubes to insure that they are not contaminated during the inoculating procedure.

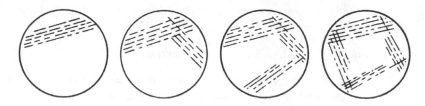

Figure 2.3 The Streak Plate. Microbes are quickly brushed or streaked across the cell-culture medium so as to allow cell growth on the plate surface.

Replica plating—velvet disks are used to pick up some of the cells from colonies on an agar medium. The disk is used to imprint the cells onto other agar plates that either lack nutrients or contain substances that select against (i.e., kill or stop the growth of) mutant cells. Colonies that do not grow on the replica plates are used to identify which of the colonies on the original plate contain the mutant cells. This technique is also used to identify clones.

Some organisms, including many parasites, cannot be cultured in synthetic media, but must be cultured in living cells. Sometimes this can be accomplished with cell or tissue culture techniques; in other cases, the organism must be cultured in a living animal.

Culture methods for molds and yeasts are similar to those used for bacteria.

2.5.3   Serial Dilutions of Broths

Proper dilution of cultures is important for accurate enumeration of microorganisms. One milliliter (ml) of a bacterial suspension is added to 9 ml sterile water, resulting in a 1:10 dilution of the original sample. One milliliter of the 1:10 dilution is added to 9 ml sterile water, yielding a 1:100 dilution. The number of bacteria are reduced one-tenth each time. The process can be repeated to achieve 1:1,000, 1:10,000, 1:100,000 dilutions, etc. The number of cells in 1 ml of the original sample is equal to the number of cells (or colonies) counted, multiplied by the reciprocal of the dilution.

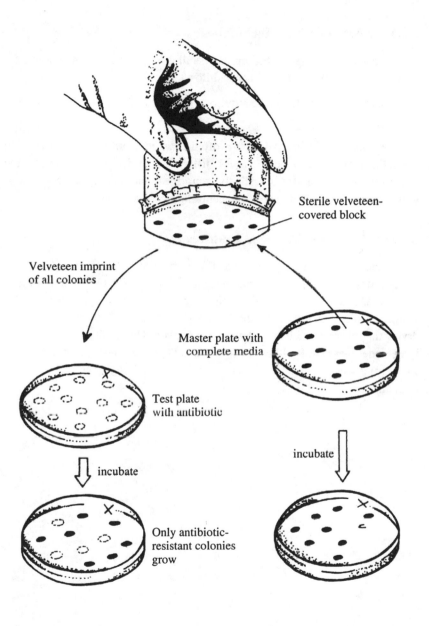

Sterile velveteen-covered block

Velveteen imprint of all colonies

Master plate with complete media

Test plate with antibiotic

incubate

incubate

Only antibiotic-resistant colonies grow

Figure 2.4 Replica Plating

2.5.4 Special Culture Techniques

Mycobacterium leprae, the leprosy bacillus, requires low temperatures for growth and has been cultured in armadillos.

Rickettsias and chlamydiae require a living host cell to complete their life cycles.

Carbon dioxide incubators are often used in laboratories to maintain specialized carbon dioxide levels for different organisms. For example, the organisms responsible for brucellosis, gonorrhea, and meningococcal meningitis require high carbon dioxide concentrations in culture.

2.5.5 Preserving Bacterial Cultures

Bacterial cultures may be stored for short or long terms. For short-term storage (days to weeks), refrigeration is the method used most often. For long-term storage (weeks to years), the rapid deep freezing of the specimen, usually with liquid nitrogen, is used. **Lyophilization** is also used, which involves freeze-drying the specimen such that all water is removed. The result of lyophilization is a powder material. Both freeze-drying and lyophilization allow for the storage of microbial cultures for years without loss of viability or an accumulation of mutations.

CHAPTER 3

Survey of Microorganisms

3.1 Prokaryotes and Eukaryotes

Prokaryotes are organisms that lack a membrane-bound nucleus and membrane-bound organelles. All members of the Kingdom Monera are prokaryotes.

Eukaryotes are organisms in which the DNA (deoxyribonucleic acid) is enclosed within a membrane-bound nucleus; organelles are membrane-bound as well. All of the Protista, Fungi, Plantae, and Animalia are eukaryotes. Eukaryotic cells are usually larger and more complex than prokaryotic cells. Microscopic eukaryotes fall within the realm of microbiology. There are other characteristic differences between these two cell types (see Table 3.1); however, they are similar in chemical reactions and composition, e.g., both contain DNA and RNA (ribonucleic acid), plasma membranes, and ribosomes.

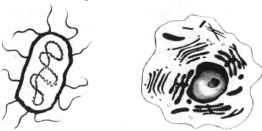

Figure 3.1 Typical Prokaryotic Cell, Left, and Eukaryotic Cell

Table 3.1 Comparison of Prokaryotes and Eukaryotes

Characteristic or Process	Prokaryotes	Eukaryotes
Membrane-bound organelles (including nucleus, mitochondria, chloroplast)	Absent	Present
Golgi apparatus	Absent	Present
Endoplasmic reticulum	Absent	Present
Chlorophylls, when present	Pigments in cytoplasm	Pigments located in membrane-bound chloroplast
Location of respiratory enzymes	Cell membrane	Mitochondria
Ribosomes	Small (70S*), free in cytoplasm	Larger (80S), bound to membranes within the cytoplasm
Plasma membrane	Fluid mosaic	Fluid mosaic with sterols
Cell wall, when present	Generally complex, contains peptidoglycan	Generally simple, may contain cellulose, chitin. Does not contain peptidoglycan
Flagellar protein	Flagellin	Tubulin
Cilia	Absent	Present
Mitosis	Lacking	Present
Genetic information	Single chromosome, without associated proteins, located in area called the nucleosome	Multiple chromosomes, with associated proteins, located in membrane-bound nucleus
Extrachromosomal DNA	In plasmids	In organelles such as the mitochondria and chloroplasts

*S is a sedimentation constant roughly proportional to MW.

3.2 Bacteria

Bacteria are unicellular prokaryotes, ranging in diameter from about 0.20 to 2.0 μm. Bacteria reproduce by binary fission.

Until an official system of classification can be agreed upon, bacteriologists turn to *Bergey's Manual of Systematic Bacteriology* for practical classification of bacteria. *Bergey's Manual* was first published in 1923 as *Bergey's Manual of Determinative Bacteriology*. In *Bergey's Manual*, bacteria are identified and grouped on the basis of a number of characteristics, including: morphology (size, shape, arrangement), staining characteristics (gram-positive, gram-negative, acid-fast), nutritional requirements, growth characteristics, physical requirements (e.g., temperature and pH optima), biochemistry, genetics, spore-forming ability, type of movement, pathogenicity, antigen/antibody testing, DNA hybridization, and GC (guanine/cytosine) ratio.

The primary **bacterial shapes** are **bacillus** (rodlike), **coccus** (spherical), and **curved**. Bacilli in pairs are known as diplobacilli; in chains, they are called

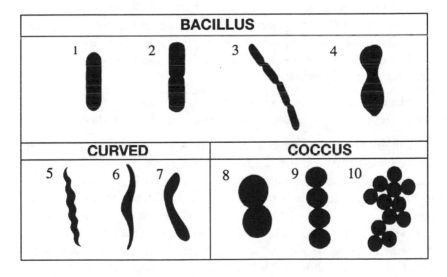

1	Single	5	Spirochete	8	Diplococcus
2	Diplobacillus (pair)	6	Spirillum	9	Streptococcus
3	Streptobacillus (chain)	7	Vibrio	10	Staphylococcus
4	Cocco-bacillus				

Figure 3.2 Primary Bacterial Shapes

19

streptobacilli. Coccobacillus are bacilli shaped so short and wide that they resemble cocci. Pairs of cocci are diplococci; chains, streptococci. Irregular aggregations are staphylococci. Among the curved types are the **spirillum**, a flexible spiral, the **spirochete,** which forms a helix, and the comma-shaped **vibrio.** Bacteria that can assume several shapes are called **pleomorphic.**

3.2.1 Bacterial Anatomy

Structures **external** to the cell wall include the glycocalyx, flagella, and pili.

Glycocalyx—a polysaccharide-containing structure that functions in attachment to solid surfaces, preventing desiccation, and protection. It consists of a **capsule** and/or a **slime layer.**

Bacterial flagella—long, thin, filamentous structures composed of the protein **flagellin** that function in cell motility. Bacterial flagella originate in the cytoplasm at a basal body. Cells with one flagellum are monotrichous, those with many are multitrichous, and those lacking flagella are atrichous. Cells may differ in flagellar arrangement as well as in the number of flagella. [**Axial filaments (endoflagella)** are *subsurface* structures unique to spirochetes. They are similar to flagella, but wrap around the cell and cause the cell to move with a characteristic corkscrew-like motion.]

Flagella enable bacteria to move toward favorable conditions (**positive chemotaxis)** or away from unfavorable conditions (**negative chemotaxis).**

Pili are tiny hollow projections composed of a protein known as **pilin.** They are much smaller than flagella (visible only with electron microscopy or special techniques) and are not involved in cell motility. There are two kinds of pili: F pili, which function in the exchange of DNA during bacterial conjugation, and fimbriae, which are shorter than F pili and function in attaching the cell to other surfaces, enhancing colonization. Pili can affect infectivity—e.g., *Neisseria gonorrhoeae* with pili are highly infectious, but those lacking pili usually do not cause disease. Pili also serve as receptor sites for viruses.

The **cell wall** surrounds the plasma membrane and serves to protect the cell from changes in osmotic pressure, anchor flagella, maintain cell shape, and control transport of molecules into and out of the cell.

The typical **bacterial cell wall** is composed primarily of **peptidoglycan,** which is a polymer of two simple amino acid sugars: N-acetylglucosamine (NAG, gluNAc) and N-acetylmuramic acid (NAM, murNAc). Additional constituents include the **porins** and the **channel proteins**, which function in transport of molecules through the cell wall.

In addition to peptidoglycan, the cell walls of **gram-positive** bacteria also contain **teichoic acids**, polysaccharides that serve as attachment sites for bacteriophages (bacterial viruses).

Gram-negative cell walls are multilayered with a lipoprotein-lipopolysaccharide-phospholipid outer membrane external to the relatively thin peptidoglycan layer. This outer membrane protects the cell from antibiotics (e.g., penicillin) and enzymes (e.g., lysozyme).

Due to these differences in their cell walls, gram-negative and gram-positive cells differ in their susceptibility to lysozyme (an enzyme that attacks bacterial cell walls). The walls of gram-positive organisms are completely destroyed by lysozyme—the resultant structure, a cell with very little or no cell wall, is called a **protoplast**. The walls of gram-negative bacteria are more resistant and are not completely destroyed—the resultant cell, with a partial cell wall, is a **spheroplast**. Neither protoplasts nor spheroplasts are protected from osmotic lysis.

Bacteria of the genus *Mycoplasma* do not have cell walls.

L forms are bacteria that have defective cell walls.

Archaebacteria have cell walls that lack peptidoglycan and consist of pseudomurein.

Structures **interior** to the cell wall include the plasma membrane, the cytoplasm, and cytoplasmic constituents such as DNA, ribosomes, and inclusions.

The **plasma membrane** is a dynamic, selectively permeable membrane enclosing the cytoplasm. It is located between the cell wall and the cytoplasm, and it regulates movement of substances, including water, into and out of the cell. The plasma membrane consists of a phospholipid bilayer containing both integral and peripheral proteins. This type of membrane is called a **fluid mosaic** and is found in both prokaryotic and eukaryotic cells.

The **DNA** of prokaryotes consists of a single, circular chromosome located in an area of the cytoplasm known as the nuclear area or nucleoid. Sometimes

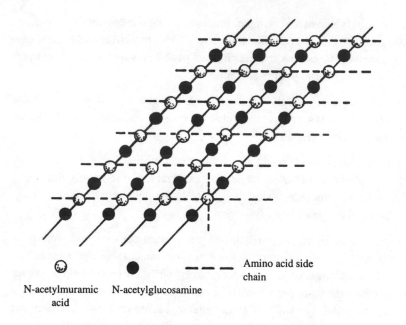

N-acetylmuramic acid   N-acetylglucosamine   Amino acid side chain

The molecules of peptidoglycan, above, show alternation of two different simple amino acid sugars that are held by amino acid side chains.

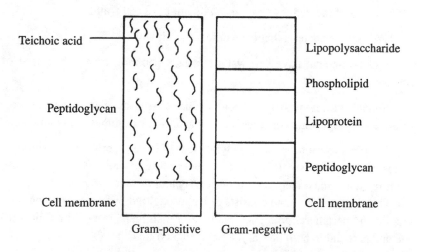

Teichoic acid

Peptidoglycan

Cell membrane

Gram-positive   Gram-negative

Lipopolysaccharide

Phospholipid

Lipoprotein

Peptidoglycan

Cell membrane

Figure 3.3 Gram-positive and Gram-negative Cell Walls. Each bacterial cell wall differs by structure and type of peptidoglycan present.

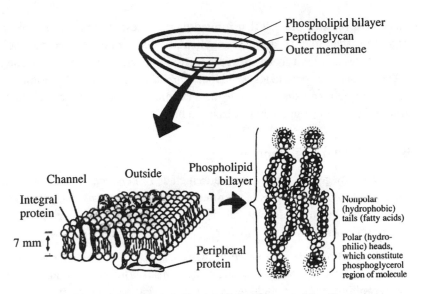

Figure 3.4 Fluid-Mosaic Model of the Plasma Membrane

bacteria contain additional small DNA circles known as **plasmids**. Plasmids are not chromosomes and do not contain essential genetic information. They sometimes carry genes for antibiotic resistance and are a means for the spread of antibiotic resistance among bacterial populations.

Inclusions are accumulations of reserve deposits. Membrane-enclosed inclusions (**vesicles**) comprise carboxysomes, gas vacuoles, and lipid inclusions. Those without membranes are called **granules**.

Metachromatic granules are large inclusions, so called because they stain red with methylene blue. These granules are also referred to as **volutin granules** and are an indication of inorganic phosphate storage. These types of granules are commonly found in algae, fungi, protozoa, and bacteria. They are characteristic of *Corynebacterium diphtheriae*, the cause of diphtheria. **Polysaccharide granules** are reddish-brown or blue when stained with iodine. The reddish-brown stain is an indication of glycogen inclusions. The blue stain is an indication of starch inclusions. *Thiobacillus* (spp.) or "sulfur bacteria" obtain energy by oxidizing sulfur and contain **sulfur granules**.

During periods of adverse conditions, some bacteria form heat-resistant resting cells known as **endospores** (within the cell that formed them) or

exospores (outside the cell that formed them). These dormant structures are highly resistant to heat, desiccation, chemical disinfection, stains, and radiation. Spores are not a means of reproduction in bacteria as they are in fungi; rather, a bacterial spore helps *the cell that produced it* to survive. Germination is the return to the vegetative state once conditions have improved. **Cysts** are resistant to drying, but are not resistant to heat.

3.2.2   Bacterial Taxonomy

Important genera of the **spirochetes** include *Treponema, Borrelia,* and *Leptospira*. These are examples of gram-negative, aquatic animal parasites. They are distinguished by their long, slender shape and crawling movements due to an axial filament.

Members of the genera *Spirillum, Azospirillum, Campylobacter,* and *Bdellovibrio* are found in soil and aquatic environments. This group of **aerobic/microaerophilic, motile, helical/vibroid, gram-negative bacteria** include nitrogen-fixing bacteria.

Nonmotile or rarely motile gram-negative bacteria are not pathogenic. **Gram-negative, aerobic rods and cocci,** such as the genera *Pseudomonas, Legionella, Neisseria, Brucella, Bordatella, Francisella, Rhizobium, Agrobacterium, Acetobacter, Gluconobacter,* and *Zooglea,* are important organisms to medicine, industry, and the environment.

Many important pathogens, including Enterobacteriaceae *(Escherichia, Salmonella, Shigella, Klebsiella, Yersinia, Enterobacter),* Vibrionaceae *(Vibrio),* Pasteurellas *(Hemophilus, Gardnerella,* and *Pasteurella),* belong to the group of **facultative anaerobic, gram-negative rods.**

Escherichia coli (E. coli) is not usually considered a pathogen. However, it can be responsible for urinary tract infection, diarrhea, and very serious foodborne diseases.

The obligate anaerobes *Bacteroides* (spp.) and *Fusobacterium* (spp.) are part of the group of **anaerobic, gram-negative, straight, curved, or helical rods.** *Bacteroides* (spp.) are commonly found in the intestinal tract of humans and the rumens of ruminants, and *Fusobacterium* (spp.) are found in the gums.

Desulfovibrio is an important genus of the **dissimilatory sulfate-reducing or sulfur-reducing bacterial group.** This group of bacteria is important ecologically.

Veillonella (spp.) are nonmotile **anaerobic, gram-negative cocci.** These are associated with dental plaque.

Members of the genera *Coxiella,* as well as *Rickettsia* and *Chlamydia,* are important pathogens of arthropods and animals. *Coxiella burnetii* causes Q fever. Species of *Rickettsia* cause typhus and Rocky Mountain spotted fever. Certain species of *Chlamydia* cause trachoma, nongonococcal urethritis, psittacosis, and mild pneumonia.

Mycoplasmas lack cell walls; thus, they are penicillin resistant. They are parasites of animals, plants, and insects and are gram-negative bacteria. *M. pneumoniae* causes walking pneumonia. *Spiroplasma* (spp.) are parasites of plant-feeding insects. Species of *Ureaplasma* may be involved in urinary tract infections. *Thermoplasma* (spp.) are not pathogenic.

Gram-positive cocci include *Staphylococcus, Streptococcus, Lactococcus,* and *Enterococcus* and may be pathogenic. The most important species of *Staphylococcus* is *S. aureus,* which is the cause of toxic shock syndrome. *S. aureus* produces exotoxin, which increases this organism's pathogenicity. Streptococci cause diseases such as scarlet fever, pharyngitis, and pneumococcal pneumonia. Lactococci are important in the dairy industry, and enterococci are occasional pathogens.

Endospore-forming, gram-positive rods and cocci are important in industry and medicine. *Bacillus anthracis* is a rod-shaped member of this group and causes anthrax. Clostridia, also rod shaped, cause tetanus, botulism, diarrhea, and gas gangrene. *Sporosarcina* (spp.) are saprophytic soil cocci.

Lactobacillus is a part of the group of **regular, nonsporing, gram-positive bacteria.** Lactobacilli have important uses in the food industry and are found in the human vagina, intestinal tract, and mouth. *Listeria monocytogenes* is a common contaminant of food products and is a pathogenic member of this group of bacteria.

The bacterial group of **irregular, nonsporing, gram-positive rods** contains human pathogens, including *Corynebacterium, Propionibacterium,* and *Actinomyces. Corynebacterium diphtheriae* causes diphtheria. *Propionibacterium acnes* may be involved in acne. *Actinomyces israelii* causes actinomycosis.

Mycobacteria include the important pathogens *Mycobacterium tuberculosis* and *M. leprae.* Members of this group are aerobic, nonsporing, nonmotile rods.

Some **nocardioforms** are aerobic, gram-positive bacteria. *Nocardia* and *Rhodococcus* are members of this group.

Members of the **gliding, sheathed and budding, and/or appendaged bacteria** include *Hyphomicrobium* and *Caulobacter.* Appendaged bacteria are characterized by the presence of a **prostheca** or protrusion. *Caulobacter* is an appendaged bacterium. Gliding, nonfruiting bacteria include *Cytophaga* and *Beggiatoa* and are characterized by their gliding motion. Gliding, fruiting bacteria include *myxobacterium*. *Hyphomicrobium* is a budding bacterium that does not reproduce by fission. *Sphaerotilus natans* are sheathed bacteria important in sewage treatment.

Nitrifying and sulfur-oxidizing aerobic **chemoautotrophic bacteria** include *Nitrosomonas, Nitrobacter,* and *Thiobacillus.* Members of this group are consequential in agriculture and in the environment.

Archaeobacteria, including *Methanobacterium, Halobacterium* and *Sulfolobus,* can be both gram-positive or gram-negative. Members of this group are characterized by the unusual environments in which they live. *Halobacteria* require high sodium chloride concentrations in their environment. *Sulfolobus* live at temperatures around 70°C, pH of 2, and in high sulfur concentrations. *Methanobacteria* are used in sewage treatment to produce methane from hydrogen and carbon dioxide.

Phototrophic bacteria are photosynthetic, gram-negative bacteria that use light as a source of energy. Green and purple sulfur bacteria are **anoxygenic** bacteria that do not produce oxygen during photosynthesis. *Anabaena* are cyanobacteria and are oxygenic phototrophic bacteria.

Actinomycetes are filamentous, gram-positive bacteria, which include *Streptomyces, Frankia,* and *Micromonospora.* Some species of *Streptomyces* produce many antibiotics, which are used commercially.

3.3 The Eukaryotic Cell

The most characteristic feature of a eukaryotic cell is the presence of membrane-bound organelles, especially the nucleus to which the name refers (*eu*—meaning true, and *karyon*—for nucleus).

Structures **external** to the cell wall or glycocalyx include flagella and cilia. Not all eukaryotic cells contain flagella or cilia. When present, eukaryotic flagella and cilia are composed of **microtubules**, which appear in a "nine pairs + two pairs" (9 + 2) arrangement. Eukaryotic flagella are composed of a protein called tubulin. Flagella are long and thin and few in number; cilia are short and numerous.

When present (in fungi and some plant cells), **eukaryotic cell walls** generally consist of either chitin or cellulose. The cell walls of yeast are composed of glucan and mannan.

Animal cells do not have a cell wall. The **glycocalyx** serves to strengthen the cell and provide a means of attachment.

In protozoans, other protective structures such as **pellicles** and **tests** may be produced.

The **eukaryotic plasma membrane** is similar to that of prokaryotes; i.e., it is composed of a phospholipid bilayer with associated proteins (the **fluid mosaic** model). Additionally, the eukaryotic plasma membrane contains sterols and attached carbohydrates. (Sterols are absent in prokaryotes, with the exception of *Mycoplasma*.) The eukaryotic plasma membrane functions in the transport of molecules into and out of the cell.

The **cytoplasm** of a eukaryotic cell contains DNA, ribosomes, inclusions, organelles (e.g., nucleus, mitochondria, chloroplasts, Golgi apparatus), and a cytoskeleton.

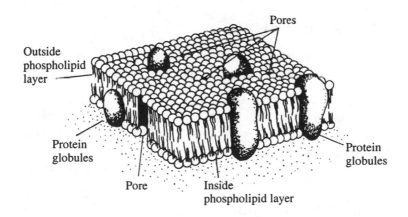

Figure 3.5 Schematic Depiction of a Typical Cell Membrane

27

The **DNA** of eukaryotes is arranged in paired chromosomes, with associated proteins (histones). It is located in a membrane-bound organelle called the nucleus.

There are two theories regarding the **evolution of cellular organelles**. According to the **endosymbiont theory**, organelles evolved from a symbiosis in which some prokaryotes lived inside other prokaryotes. Supporters of this hypothesis cite the occurrence of 70S ribosomes in both mitochondria and chloroplasts, and the fact that these organelles multiply by fission—both characteristics of prokaryotic cells. Eukaryotic cells contain larger ribosomes (80S) and undergo mitotic division.

According to the **autogenous hypothesis**, organelles evolved from the plasma membrane. Organelles that seem to support this theory include the nucleus and the Golgi apparatus.

3.3.1   Algae

Algae is a catchall term for photosynthetic aquatic organisms, both unicellular and multicellular. Depending on its pigments and structures, an alga can be classified as either a plant or a protist. Algae are the primary energy producers in aquatic environments and are important in several food chains. They vary greatly in size (from microscopic to greater than 60 m in length), and also in shape and organization. Reproduction may be either sexual or asexual (fragmentation, division by splitting, unicellular spores).

3.3.1.1   Classification of Algae

Six algal divisions are recognized: the unicellular Chlorophyta, Chrysophyta, Euglenophyta, and Pyrrophyta, and the multicellular Phaeophyta and Rhodophyta.

Brown algae (Phaeophyta) or kelp can grow to be 50 meters in length. Brown algae also have very fast growth rates. Algin is harvested from the cell wall of brown algae and is used as a thickener in ice cream and cake decorations. It also has nonfood uses and is used in the production of rubber tires and hand lotion.

Red algae (Rhodophyta) have delicate branches called **thalli**. Agar is produced by red algae. Carrageenan is harvested from a red algae called Irish moss and is used as a thickener in evaporated milk and ice cream. Some may also be used medicinally as antihelminthics, as antidiarrheals, and in cancer chemotherapy.

Green algae (Chlorophyta) are thought to be the ancestors of terrestrial plants. Filamentous green algae form pond scum.

Diatoms (Chrysophyta) have complex cell walls composed of two halves that overlap like a petri dish containing pectin and silica and have distinctive patterns. In diatoms, energy is stored in the form of oil (crude oil). Deposits of dead diatoms form diatomaceous earth, which is used in detergents, abrasive polishes, and paint removers and as a filtering and insulating agent.

Dinoflagellates (Pyrrophyta) or **plankton** are free-floating organisms whose cell walls contain cellulose and silica. Eighty percent of the world's oxygen is produced by plankton. *Gonyaulax* is a dinoflagellate, which produces neurotoxins (saxitoxin), which cause paralytic shellfish poisoning. The shellfish are not harmed by the toxin, but it accumulates within the shellfish, making them highly toxic to vertebrates that eat them. These are also responsible for red tides, which are large blooms of dinoflagellates coloring the ocean red. Diatoms and other plankton are responsible for the supply of petroleum.

Euglenoids (Euglenophyta) are unicellular, flagellated organisms characterized by a **pellicle,** or semirigid plasma membrane; a **red eye spot (stigma),** or carotenoid organelle; a cytosome, used for digestion; and one or two **preemergent flagella** for locomotion.

3.3.2 Fungi

The **fungi** (molds, yeast, and mushrooms) are nonmotile, nonphotosynthetic eukaryotes. They absorb nutrients from their environment. A few species are **parasitic**, but most are **saprophytic**, absorbing nutrients from dead organic matter. Fungi are important ecologically; they are, along with bacteria, the decomposers of the world. They are important economically as well, especially in the area of food spoilage. Fungal cell walls generally contain chitin, although yeast cell walls contain the complex polysaccharides glucan and mannan.

A **mushroom** consists of a vegetative structure known as a **thallus,** which is composed of filaments called **hyphae.** A **mycelium** is a mass of hyphae. **Molds** consist of long chains of cells that occasionally form hyphae; they reproduce by spores.

Yeasts are unicellular fungi that reproduce asexually by budding. Buds that do not separate from the mother cell form **pseudohyphae. Dimorphic** fungi appear yeastlike at 37°C, moldlike at 25°C. Some yeast have pili on their cell walls. These structures, similar to the pili of bacteria, may be involved in the sexual reproduction of yeast.

3.3.2.1 Classification of Fungi

Although fungi reproduce both sexually and asexually, they are divided into two groups, the Ascomycetes and the **Basidiomycetes,** on the basis of their type of sexual reproduction. In a third group of fungi, however, the **Fungi Imperfecti,** the sexual stage has never been observed.

Deuteromycota (imperfect fungi) are a phylum of fungi that have not yet been observed to produce sexual spores. Members of this phylum, therefore, cannot be classified. However, once sexual spores are observed, the organisms may be classified.

Zygomycota (conjugation fungi) include *Rhizopus nigricans,* the common black bread mold, which produces asexual sporangiospores and sexual **zygospores.** Zygospores are large, surrounded by a thick wall, and can remain dormant if the environment is too harsh for growth.

Ascomycota (sac fungi) produce **conidiospores,** which produce a spore dust when disturbed. The sexual spore is classified as an ascospore because the spores are produced in an ascus or saclike structure. *Eupenicillium* is a member of this phylum. *Claviceps purpurea* is a parasitic member of this class parasitizing rye and other grasses and causing the disease ergot.

Basidiomycota (club fungi) include mushrooms. These organisms produce **basidiospores** and asexual conidiospores. Basidiospores form on a base pedestal, the **basidium.** They are used as food and help to decompose plant debris.

3.3.2.2 Fungal Disease

Mycosis is the term for any **fungal infection** or **disease** and can include systemic mycoses, subcutaneous mycoses, cutaneous mycoses, and superficial mycoses. Fungi may be important in opportunistic infections of debilitated or immunosuppressed patients. Examples of opportunistic mycoses are mucormycosis, aspergillosis, candidiasis, and thrush. Mucormycosis is caused by *Rhizopus* and *Mucor.* Aspergillosis is caused by inhalation of *Aspergillus* spores.

Candidiasis is caused by *Candida albicans*. Thrush causes an inflammation of the mouth and throat.

3.3.2.3 Commercially Important Fungi

Saccharomyces cerevisiae is a **yeast** important in the food industry. It is used in the production of bread and wine. *Trichoderma* produces the enzyme cellulase used in the production of fruit juice. *Taxomyces* is a **fungus** that produces taxol, an anticancer drug. *Phytophthora infestans* is the potato fungus responsible for the potato crop failure in Ireland in the 1800s. Dutch elm disease is caused by *Ceratocystis ulmi*.

3.3.3 Lichens and Slime Molds

The lichens and slime molds are not easily classified.

A **lichen** is the result of a symbiosis between an alga and a fungus. The fungus provides structural support and the alga provides nutrients. Lichens are able to occupy habitats that would not be suitable for either the fungus or the alga alone.

Slime molds are sometimes classified as fungi, sometimes as protozoans. Most are saprophytic, but some are parasitic. They exist in two forms: cellular and acellular.

An **acellular,** or **plasmodial,** slime mold is a multinucleated mass of protoplasm that engulfs bacteria and organic matter as it moves along.

Cellular slime molds ingest bacteria by phagocytosis; they resemble amoebas.

3.3.4 Protozoans

Protozoans are unicellular eukaryotes. Most are motile, microscopic, and heterotrophic, feeding on bacteria or particulate organic matter. There are thousands of species, about two dozen of which cause disease in humans.

Lacking a cell wall, protozoans employ such protective structures as **pellicles** (a strong outer covering found in ciliates and some amoebas), **tests** (shells of calcium carbonate or silica), and **trichocysts** (specialized defense organelles). Some protozoans also form **cysts**, resting stages with thick resistant coverings.

Trophozoite—the active feeding stage of a protozoan (the term is used for both free-living and parasitic protozoans).

Protozoans reproduce **sexually** by conjugation, autogamy, or syngamy; and **asexually** by budding, binary fission, multiple fission, or plasmotomy.

Conjugation involves the transfer of DNA between cells via a temporary connection.

Autogamy is a modification of conjugation.

Syngamy is the fusion of two different types of sex cells.

Plasmotomy is splitting into two or more multinucleated cells.

3.3.4.1 Classification of Protozoans

Protozoans are classified according to their mode of locomotion. Those using whiplike **flagella** for locomotion belong to the Mastigophora; those using hairlike **cilia** are the Ciliates; those moving via **pseudopodia** (amoeboid movement) belong to the Sarcodina; and those lacking a means of locomotion as adults belong to the Sporozoa (all sporozoans are obligate parasites).

Sarcomastigophora is the phylum of protozoans that consists of organisms that use either pseudopods or flagella as a form of locomotion. For example, *Naegleria* and other species use both forms of locomotion.

Sarcodina is the subphylum of the amoeboflagellates that use pseudopods or cytoplasmic projections to move. *Entamoeba histolytica* causes amoebic dysentery, which is endemic in many parts of the world. Some amoebas, such as *Acanthamoeba,* can pass through the blood-brain barrier.

Some parasitic amoebae that use flagellae are called **flagellates.** Among them are *Giardia lamblia,* which causes intestinal infections, *Trichomonas vaginalis,* which causes a genitourinary infection, and *Trypanosoma,* which causes African sleeping sickness *(T. brucei gambiense)* and Chagas' disease *(T. cruzi).* This phylum of flagellates is **Mastigophora.**

Ciliates use cilia for locomotion (Ciliophora) and to propel food towards the mouth. Ciliates are **multinucleate** with both a macronucleus and one or more micronuclei. A parasitic ciliate is *Balantidium coli,* which causes dysentery.

Apicomplexa is the phylum that consists of mature, nonmotile organisms with complex life cycles. *Plasmodium,* which causes malaria, is an example of an **apicomplexan.** *Toxoplasma gondii,* which spends its life cycle in domestic cats, can cause congenital infections in pregnant women.

Cryptosporidium causes respiratory and diarrheal diseases in immunosuppressed patients. *Pneumocystis carinii* causes pneumonia.

Microspora is a phylum of protozoans that are obligatory intracellular parasites responsible for chronic diarrhea and keratoconjunctivitis. The human pathogen is *Nosema* and is commonly found in AIDS patients. *Nosema locustae* is used in residual control of rangeland grasshoppers.

3.3.5 Animal Microbes—Helminths

Certain stages in the life cycles of **helminths** are microscopic. Helminths include the Platyhelminthes, or flatworms (e.g., the liver fluke), and the nematodes, or roundworms (e.g., hookworm).

3.3.5.1 Classification of Helminths

The phylum **Platyhelminthes (flatworms)** contains the trematodes and cestodes. Members of this phylum have incomplete digestive systems. These flatworms have only one opening through which both nutrients and waste products flow.

The **trematodes** are **flukes** characterized by a ventral or oral sucker by which the organism holds on to its host and by a **cuticle,** or nonliving covering, through which it absorbs food. *Clonorchis sinensis* is an Asian liver fluke and causes clonorchiasis. *Schistosoma* is a fluke that infects humans through the skin and causes the disease schistosomiasis.

Paragonimus westermani is a lung fluke. The adult fluke lives in the lung and lays eggs in the sputum of the bronchi. Sputum is swallowed and eggs are excreted by the human host. The eggs must then enter water to complete the life cycle. The **miracidium** develops within the egg. The secondary hosts are snails that live in the water. In the snail the miracidium develops into a **redia,** which produces **rediae** by asexual reproduction. The rediae develop into **cercaria,** which then find a tertiary host, a crayfish. **Metacercaria** develop from cercaria in the crayfish. When the crayfish are eaten by humans, the metacercaria find their way to the lungs, where they develop into an adult fluke.

Cestodes are **tapeworms.** These are intestinal parasites, which may attach to their host by sucker or by hook. The digestive system is absent in these organisms. The head is called the **scolex,** which contains the sucker or hook, and the body consists of segments called **proglottids.** Each body segment is hermaphroditic.

Taenia saginata is the beef tapeworm, whose adult form lives in the human intestine and can reach lengths of 6 meters. Their eggs are ingested by grazing cattle. The eggs hatch in the bovine intestine, and the larval form migrates to the muscle where these encyst as **cysticerci.** The cysticerci can be ingested by humans when they consume the contaminated meat.

Taenia solium is the porcine tapeworm. The hosts of this tapeworm are also humans. Cysticercosis is a disease characterized by human-to-human transmission of eggs, where the cysticerci encyst in the brain of the human host.

The phylum **Nematoda,** or **roundworms,** consists of organisms with complete digestive systems. Some nematodes are free living in soil while others are parasites and require a host. Male roundworms have one or two spicules on their posterior ends that are used to guide the male sperm to the genital pore on the female. There are two types of roundworms, those whose eggs are infective and those whose larvae are infective.

Enterobius vermicularis, or pinworms, may complete their entire life cycle within a human host. Eggs are laid on the perianal skin of the host and are transmitted through clothing or bedding. The adult form of *Ascaris lumbricoides* inhabits the intestines of humans, pigs, and horses. The eggs are transmitted through feces and are ingested by hosts.

Necator americanus is the adult hookworm. The adult form is found in the small intestine of humans, and eggs are found in feces. The eggs hatch in soil, and the larval form may infect a host via the skin. *Trichinella spiralis,* which causes trichinosis, is transmitted via undercooked pork meat. The larval form is encysted in this meat. The female does not lay eggs; instead, eggs develop within the female. The female gives live birth.

3.4   Viruses

Depending on one's point of view, viruses are either extremely complex nonliving entities or extremely simple forms of life. Capable of parasitizing every kind of life, they have no nutritional patterns of their own. They do not grow. They have no cellular structures. Their only observable activity is nucleic acid replication, and this can be accomplished only within a living cell. They are not assigned to any kingdom.

The mature virus particle—the **virion**—consists of nucleic acid (either RNA or DNA) and a protein sheath (the **capsid**), and can transfer its nucleic acid among host cells. It may or may not have an **envelope**. Enveloped viruses may have spikes that project from the surface and appear to be involved in the process of viral attachment to host cells.

The viral life cycle consists of both intra- and extracellular phases. The usual sequence of events is **attachment** to the host cell, **penetration** of the host cell, **uncoating** of the virion, **manufacture** of viral parts (under direction of the viral genome but carried out using the host's machinery, proteins, and energy), **assembly** of new virus particles, and **release** of new viruses.

Virus classification is based on morphology (including size and shape), structure, chemical and physical characteristics (especially nucleic acid chemistry and capsid organization), mode of replication, and host range.

Viruses are very small: 20–300 nm.

The major viral shapes can be described as **icosahedral** (e.g., herpes and polio viruses), **helical** (e.g., rabies, tobacco mosaic), and **complex** (see Figure 3.6).

Host range—the range of host cells in which a virus can multiply. Categories include animal viruses (e.g., chicken pox and smallpox in humans, rabies in dogs), plant viruses (e.g., tobacco mosaic virus), bacterial viruses (bacteriophages), or cyanophyte viruses (cyanophages). A particular virus can usually infect only a few species within the more general host categories.

Animal viruses may contain either RNA or DNA; however, most plant viruses contain RNA. **Plant viruses**, usually polyhedral or helical, can produce both internal and external effects and have an economic impact on agriculture.

Viroids are extremely small, low molecular weight RNA, infectious agents found mainly in plant diseases. Other so-called "small RNAs" involved in disease include satellite viruses, satellite RNAs, and defective interfering particles.

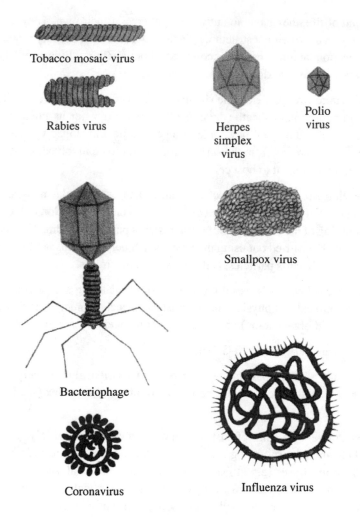

Tobacco mosaic virus

Rabies virus

Herpes simplex virus

Polio virus

Smallpox virus

Bacteriophage

Coronavirus

Influenza virus

Figure 3.6 Shapes of Viruses

3.4.1 Bacteriophages

Bacteriophages contain either RNA or DNA. Some have a taillike structure through which they inject their nucleic acid into the bacterial host cell.

Bacteriophage infection follows one of two courses—lysis or lysogeny. If the infecting virus multiplies within the host cell and destroys it, the virus is said to be **lytic**, or **virulent**. On the other hand, if the virus does not replicate but rather integrates into the bacterial chromosome, the virus is said to be **temperate**, or **lysogenic**. The phage in the lysogenic cycle can spontaneously become lytic. The presence of the integrated virus, which is called a **prophage**, generally renders the cell resistant to infection by similar phages. Lysogeny does not result in the destruction of the host cell.

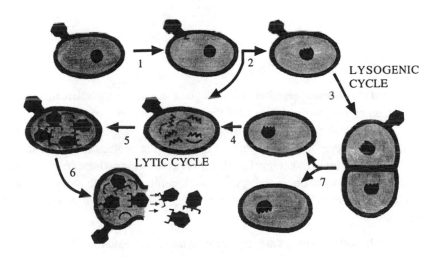

1. Phage attaches to host cell wall
2. Viral DNA is injected into cell
3. Viral DNA attaches to bacterial DNA
4. Viral DNA takes over cell and starts to reproduce
5. New protein coats are synthesized
6. Bacterium lyses and new viruses are released
7. Bacterial cell divides, producing more cells with viral DNA

Figure 3.7 Lysis and Lysogeny

CHAPTER 4

Microbial Metabolism

4.1 General Terms

All of the chemical reactions that take place in a living organism, including *anabolism* and *catabolism,* are called the **metabolism**. As part of the metabolism, **anabolism/anabolic reactions** are reactions in which energy is used to synthesize complex organic molecules from simpler molecules. These reactions require an input of energy. **Catabolism/catabolic reactions** are reactions used by organisms to obtain energy, in which complex organic molecules are oxidized and broken down into simpler molecules. These reactions release energy.

Amphibolic pathways are sequences of metabolic reactions that integrate both anabolism and catabolism. Such a pathway may either capture energy or produce substances needed by the cell.

Some reactions require a catalyst. A **catalyst** is a substance that lowers the energy of activation for a reaction. The **energy of activation** is the energy required for a reaction to take place.

4.2 Enzymes

Enzymes are proteins that catalyze chemical reactions. They are specific—

generally catalyzing only a single reaction or a group of related reactions. They are named according to their substrate (the compound they act upon) and function, e.g., glucose-6-phosphate dehydrogenase is an enzyme that functions as a dehydrogenase with glucose-6-phosphate as its substrate. Names of enzymes always end with -*ase*. Like all other proteins, enzymes can be destroyed by high temperatures; such **denatured** enzymes can no longer function as catalysts.

Enzyme activity (and thus, reaction rate) is influenced by pH, temperature (lower = slower), and concentrations of enzyme, substrate, and end product.

Enzyme + substrate → enzyme–substrate complex → enzyme + transformed substrate (product)

Some enzymes require inorganic ions, or **cofactors**. An enzyme complex consisting of the protein portion (**apoenzyme**) and a nonprotein portion (**cofactor**) is called a **holoenzyme**.

Active site—the site on the enzyme at which the substrate binds.

Enzymes (and therefore reactions) can be inhibited in a number of ways:

Competitive inhibition/competitive inhibitors—nonsubstrate molecules compete with substrate molecules for binding at the active site, directly preventing substrate binding.

Noncompetitive inhibition/noncompetitive inhibitors—nonsubstrate molecules bind to a site on the enzyme other than the active site. Binding at this **allosteric site** alters the three-dimensional shape of the enzyme and indirectly prevents substrate binding at the active site.

Feedback inhibition—the end product of the reaction binds at an allosteric site and inhibits substrate binding at the active site.

Genetic regulation—affects enzyme production (see Section 9.12).

4.3   Oxidation and Reduction

When one molecule is oxidized, another is reduced. Such reactions are known as **redox reactions**. It is the **transfer of electrons** that provides energy in a redox reaction.

Oxidation—removal of electrons.

Reduction—gain of electrons.

Cells must have electron donors, electron carriers, and electron acceptors to produce energy.

In certain metabolic reactions, energy is released and captured to form **adenosine triphosphate (ATP)** via the phosphorylation of adenosine diphosphate (ADP).

4.4 Phosphorylation

Phosphorylation—the addition of inorganic phosphate (P_i) to another molecule.

The energy required for phosphorylation may be obtained three ways: oxidative phosphorylation, photosynthetic phosphorylation, and substrate-level phosphorylation.

Oxidative phosphorylation—energy is released as electrons pass through a series of electron acceptors (the electron transport system [see section 4.5.2]) to either oxygen or some other inorganic compound. Coenzymes (e.g., FAD, NAD, NADP) are required.

Photosynthetic phosphorylation—electrons are released as light is absorbed by chlorophyll, and they subsequently pass through the electron transport system (see also section 4.7).

Substrate-level phosphorylation—energy, in the form of a high energy phosphate, is released from a substrate (e.g., a metabolic intermediate) through enzyme activity.

4.5 Carbohydrate Catabolism

The oxidation of glucose (a reduced molecule) provides energy for the cell.

Pathways for the oxidation of organic compounds (e.g., glucose) and the capture of energy in the form of ATP can be divided into three major groups. These groups differ primarily in the substance or molecule that serves as the final electron acceptor.

Fermentation—redox occurs in absence of any added electron acceptor; glucose is only partially broken down.

Aerobic respiration—glucose is completely broken down with molecular oxygen serving as the final electron acceptor.

Anaerobic respiration—an inorganic ion other than molecular oxygen (e.g., NO_3^-, SO_4^{2-}, CO_3^{2-}) serves as the final electron acceptor. Anaerobic respiration yields fewer ATP molecules than does aerobic respiration because only part of the Krebs cycle (see section 4.5.2) is operative under anaerobic conditions.

Glycolysis—the oxidation of glucose to pyruvic acid (and/or glycerol).

Alternatives to glycolysis include the **Entner-Doudoroff pathway** and the **pentose phosphate pathway**. These pathways supply sugars necessary for the synthesis of nucleotides.

4.5.1   Fermentation

Fermentation—oxidative pathways in which *organic* compounds serve as both electron acceptors and electron donors. Energy is released from sugars or other organic molecules in the absence of an added electron acceptor (i.e., an organic molecule serves as the final electron acceptor).

Fermentation produces two ATPs via substrate-level phosphorylation.

There are different kinds of fermentation. Examples include: **Alcoholic fermentation**—which produces ethanol and CO_2. **Heterolactic fermentation**—the pentose phosphate pathway is used to produce lactic acid and ethanol. **Lactic acid fermentation**—pyruvic acid is reduced to lactic acid.

4.5.2   Respiration

Respiration—oxidative pathways in which *inorganic* compounds serve as the final electron acceptors. In aerobic respiration, the final electron acceptor is molecular oxygen; in anaerobic respiration, some other inorganic molecule (e.g., nitrate, carbonate, or sulfate) acts as the final electron acceptor.

In prokaryotes, the complete oxidation of a molecule of glucose yields a total of 38 ATP molecules; in eukaryotes, 36.

41

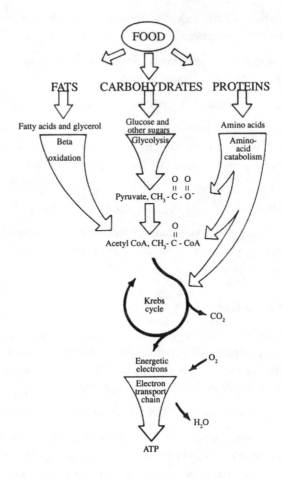

Figure 4.1 Summary: Catabolic Pathways

The steps or phases of respiration are transition, Krebs cycle, and electron transport.

Transition—following glycolysis, pyruvic acid is converted to acetyl CoA before entering the Krebs cycle. (Some texts do not treat transition separately, but rather consider it as part of the Krebs cycle.)

Krebs cycle (tricarboxylic acid [TCA] cycle, citric acid cycle)—two-carbon groups are oxidized to CO_2 and H_2O. One ATP is produced from each acetyl group. The acetyl CoA is processed so that the hydrogen atoms can be transferred to the electron transport system and oxidized for energy.

Electron transport system (electron transport chain)—a sequence of redox reactions that provide energy for the oxidative phosphorylation of three molecules of ADP to ATP. This process involves the coenzymes nicotinamide adenine dinucleotide (NAD), nicotinamide adenine dinucleotide phosphate (NADP), and flavin adenine dinucleotide (FAD), as well as carrier molecules such as flavoproteins, cytochromes, and quinones (coenzyme Q). In eukaryotes, oxidative phosphorylation takes place along the cristae of the mitochondria.

Theory of chemosmosis—as electrons move through a series of carriers or acceptors, protons being pumped across a membrane (the inner mitochondrial membrane in eukaryotes or the plasma membrane in prokaryotes) generate a **proton motive force**, the energy of which is sufficient to produce ATP.

4.6 Lipid and Protein Catabolism

Lipids are hydrolyzed into glycerol and fatty acids. Glycerol is then catabolized in glycolysis; fatty acids undergo beta oxidation to acetyl CoA, which enters the Krebs cycle.

Proteins are first broken down to amino acids, which must then be transaminated, decarboxylated, or dehydrogenated before their subsequent catabolism in either glycolysis, the Krebs cycle, or fermentation.

4.7 Photosynthesis

Photosynthesis—the utilization of light energy from the sun to synthesize carbohydrates from CO_2. The process involves conversion of the light energy into chemical energy that can be used for carbon fixation. There are two different sets of reactions in photosynthesis—the light reactions and the dark reactions (also known as the Calvin-Benson cycle).

In the **light reactions**, electrons from chlorophyll travel through an electron transport chain, producing ATP via chemosmosis. The light reactions can involve **cyclic photophosphorylation,** wherein the electrons return to chlorophyll, or **photolysis accompanied by noncyclic photophosphorylation,** wherein the electrons are used to reduce NADP; electrons from H_2O or H_2S return to chlorophyll.

In the **dark reactions**, CO_2 is reduced to synthesize carbohydrates.

4.8 Other Anabolic Pathways

Lipids are synthesized from glycerol (derived from dihydroxyacetone phosphate) and fatty acids (derived from acetyl CoA).

Proteins are synthesized from amino acids that are synthesized from intermediates in the Krebs cycle or other phases of carbohydrate metabolism.

4.9 Nutritional Modes

Autotrophs are organisms that can synthesize all of their essential biochemical compounds using *inorganic* carbon (CO_2) as their sole carbon source. All autotrophs use the same pathway for carbon fixation, i.e., the Calvin-Benson cycle (the "dark reactions" of photosynthesis). Autotrophs that use sunlight as their energy source are referred to as photosynthetic autotrophs or **photoautotrophs**; those that use inorganic compounds (e.g., hydrogen or hydrogen sulfide) as their energy source are known as chemosynthetic autotrophs or **chemoautotrophs**.

Heterotrophs are organisms that lack the ability to fix CO_2. They must obtain their carbon from an *organic* source. Some heterotrophs use light as an energy source and are known as photosynthetic heterotrophs, or **photoheterotrophs**. Chemosynthetic heterotrophs, or **chemoheterotrophs**, use organic compounds for their energy source as well as for their carbon source. Chemoheterotrophs carry out the biochemical reactions known as glycolysis, fermentation, and respiration to synthesize carbohydrates and other biochemical compounds and macromolecules.

Photosynthetic organisms oxidize water to produce oxygen and are therefore referred to as **oxygenic phototrophs**. Examples of oxygenic phototrophs are **cyanobacteria** and **algae**.

Organisms that cannot undergo photosynthesis in the presence of oxygen are **anoxygenic phototrophs**. That is, photosynthesis in these organisms does not produce oxygen. Examples of anoxygenic phototrophs are **green sulfur** and **purple sulfur bacteria**.

Table 4.1 Nutritional Modes of Organisms

	Energy Source	Carbon Source
Photoautotrophs	Light	Inorganic
Chemoautotrophs	Inorganic chemical reactions	Inorganic
Photoheterotrophs	Light	Organic
Chemoheterotrophs	Organic chemical reactions	Organic

CHAPTER 5

Transport of Molecules

5.1 Transport

Transport, or the movement of materials across the plasma membrane (or any cellular membrane), may or may not require energy expenditure from the cell. **Passive processes** (e.g., diffusion and osmosis) are those in which materials move along a concentration gradient from an area of higher concentration to an area of lower concentration and do not require energy. Conversely, **active transport** and **group translocation** involve movement of materials against a concentration gradient (i.e., from an area of lower concentration to an area of higher concentration), and they do require energy.

5.2 Simple Diffusion

Simple diffusion—materials, generally small molecules and ions, move from an area of higher concentration to an area of lower concentration until a state of equilibrium is reached (i.e., the concentration is the same on both sides of the membrane).

5.3 Osmosis

Osmosis refers specifically to the movement of water molecules across a selectively permeable membrane, from an area of higher (water) concentration to an area of lower (water) concentration until equilibrium is reached.

5.3.1 Hypotonic, Isotonic, and Hypertonic

Hypotonic environment—the concentration of solute in the extracellular medium is lower than the concentration of solute within the cell. A hypotonic environment forces the cell to expend energy via active transport or group translocation in order to move molecules into the cell against the concentration gradient. There is a danger that the cell will rupture due to the tendency of osmosis to move water into the cell under these conditions.

Isotonic environment—the concentration of solute in the extracellular medium is equal to the concentration of solute within the cell.

Hypertonic environment—the concentration of solute in the extracellular medium is greater than the concentration of solute within the cell. The cell can use diffusion processes to move molecules along the concentration gradient into the cell. Water will tend to move out of the cell by osmosis (**plasmolysis**), resulting in cell shrinkage (**crenation**).

5.4   Facilitated Diffusion

Facilitated diffusion—movement is from an area of higher concentration to one of lower concentration, but substances being transported across the membrane first combine with membrane **carrier proteins (permeases)**.

5.5   Active Transport

Active transport—**permeases** transport molecules across the membrane against the concentration gradient from an area of low concentration to an area of higher concentration. Energy (ATP) is required.

5.6   Group Translocation

Group translocation—a process unique to prokaryotes, in which energy is used to chemically alter the substance being transported. Once within the cell, the modified substance can accumulate within the cell. This process requires a high-energy phosphate compound such as ATP or PEP (phospho-enolpyruvic acid) for energy.

5.7   Endocytosis and Exocytosis

Unique to eukaryotic cells, **endocytosis** and **exocytosis** are two additional transport processes. They are important in moving large quantities of a substance. Both involve the formation of vesicles from the plasma membrane. Endocytosis is the formation of a vesicle that moves into the cell (e.g., by **phagocytosis**). Exocytosis involves the formation of vesicles that are moved out of the cell (e.g., by secretion).

CHAPTER 6

Bacterial Growth

6.1   Growth of Bacterial Populations

Growth is the orderly increase in quantity of all cellular components and structures. The growth of an individual cell leads to an increase in size and is generally followed by cell division.

Vegetative cell—one that is actively growing and dividing.

Cell division in bacteria usually occurs by **binary fission**, in which the cell divides into two new (approximately equal and identical) cells.

Cell division by **budding**, in which the new cell develops as a small outgrowth from the surface of the existing (parent) cell, occurs in some bacteria and in yeast.

Other bacteria may reproduce by fragmentation or by aerial spore formation. Although it does occur under favorable conditions as well, spore formation (**sporulation**) generally serves to allow the organism to withstand long periods of unfavorable conditions such as extreme temperatures or dryness.

Microbial growth is assayed as an increase in cell number or mass of a **population** of cells.

Generation time (doubling time)—the time it takes for an individual cell to divide or for a population of cells to double. Bacterial growth follows a **loga-**

rithmic (exponential) progression, e.g., 2 cells → 4 cells → 8 cells → 16 cells, etc.

$$\text{Generation time} = \frac{t}{3.3 \log \dfrac{B_0}{B_1}}$$

where t is the time interval between cell number measurements B_0 and B_1 during log phase growth; B_0 is the initial number of bacteria; and B_1 is the number of bacteria after time t.

When bacteria are placed in fresh, nutrient-rich medium, they exhibit four characteristic **phases of population growth**: lag phase, log phase, stationary phase, and death phase (see Figure 6.1).

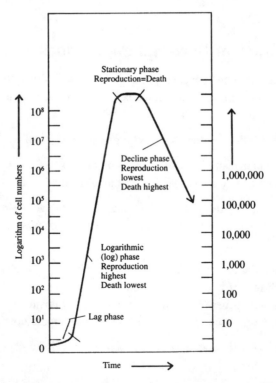

Figure 6.1 Growth of Bacterial Populations

50

Lag phase—cells are metabolically active but are not dividing. This is a period when the cells are resynthesizing enzymes, coenzymes, etc., necessary for growth and division.

Log phase—bacteria are growing and dividing at an exponential, or logarithmic, rate. This is the period of fastest growth; the generation time is maximal and constant. All nutrients and molecules needed for growth are in good supply.

Stationary phase—at this point, the medium is becoming depleted in some nutrients, and toxic quantities of waste materials may be accumulating. The number of new cells produced is offset by the number of cells that are dying; thus, the total number of viable cells remains approximately constant.

Death phase—conditions are becoming less and less conducive to cell growth. Cells are dying more rapidly than new ones are being formed, resulting in a logarithmic decrease in the number of cells.

Continuous culture—when fresh medium is continuously provided to a population of cells in log phase, the population continues to grow. In this way, a continuous culture can be maintained over long periods of time. A **chemostat** is a device that allows for the continuous addition of fresh medium.

6.2 Ways to Measure Growth of Bacterial Populations

Growth can be measured either directly or indirectly. **Direct methods** include direct microscope counts, standard plate counts, filtration, and the most probable number technique. **Indirect methods** include measurement of metabolic activity (e.g., oxygen consumption), dry weight, or turbidity (cloudiness of a suspension).

Viable count—a count that does *not* include dead cells. Standard plate counts, filtration, and most probable number are all viable count techniques. Measurement of metabolic activity, although an indirect method, also measures only viable cells. Other methods of indirect measure, as well as direct microscope counts, fail to distinguish between living and dead cells; thus, all cells, both living and dead, are included in the count.

Direct microscope counts—a measured volume of a bacterial suspension is placed on a special type of microscope slide known as a Petroff-Hauser bacterial counter (hemocytometer) and cells are counted under the microscope.

Standard plate counts are the most commonly used methods. They are based on the premise that a viable cell, when placed on the appropriate medium, will give rise to a bacterial colony; thus, cells are measured as **colony forming units** (CFUs). The formula for computing CFU is:

$$\text{CFU} = \frac{\text{number of colonies}}{\text{volume of sample}} \times \text{reciprocal of the dilution}$$

There are two standard plate count methods: the **spread plate**, in which a small sample is spread over the surface of an agar plate containing the appropriate medium, and the **pour plate**, in which the sample is mixed in with the melted agar medium before the plate is poured. Proper dilution of the sample is required as only those plates with between 30 and 300 colonies are considered valid for counting.

Filtration—a bacterial suspension, or dilution thereof, is filtered through a membrane. Cells that are retained on the membrane are resuspended and transferred to an agar plate for growth and subsequent counting of colonies.

Most probable number (MPN)—this method is based on a statistical estimation for the number of cells. It involves dilution of the sample to an estimated concentration of less than one cell per milliliter. One milliliter aliquots of the dilution are used to inoculate test tubes of fresh liquid medium, which are then observed for growth. If growth occurs, the dilution contained at least one cell. It is important to dilute the samples properly because if the sample is overly diluted, there is no growth and the count is invalid; conversely, if the sample is not diluted enough, all tubes show growth and again the count is invalid.

6.3 Physical and Chemical Requirements for Growth

For any microbe, there is a range of temperatures and pH within which it will grow. Conditions beyond those ranges may inhibit growth or even kill the organism.

Temperature—microbes vary in their range of temperature tolerance. Organisms with a narrow temperature range are said to be **stenothermal.** Those with a wide temperature range are **eurythermal.**

Psychrophiles (cryophiles) are organisms with low temperature optima, generally between 0°C and 20°C.

Mesophiles prefer mid-range temperatures, 20°C – 40°C.

Thermophiles have high temperature optima, >40°C.

Cardinal temperatures (minimum, optimum, and maximum growth temperatures) define the growth range of an organism:

Minimum growth temperature—the organism cannot grow below this temperature.

Optimum growth temperature—temperature at which it grows best/most rapidly.

Maximum growth temperature—temperature above which growth does not occur.

The **temperature range** of an organism extends from the minimum growth temperature through the maximum growth temperature.

pH—a measure of acidity or alkalinity. pH values between 5 and 9 are common in nature, and the pH optima of many organisms falls within this range. However, there are organisms that can live at a pH of as low as 0 or as high as 12. Organisms preferring low pH environments are called **acidophiles.** Generally, an organism cannot tolerate drastic changes in pH; the range of acceptable pH values is usually only about one pH unit.

Chemically, bacteria require nitrogen, carbon, and energy sources; water; vitamins and growth factors; and essential mineral salts (e.g., phosphorus, potassium, iron, sulfur).

Nitrogen (organic or inorganic)—necessary for synthesis of proteins and nucleic acids. NH_4^+, NO_3^-, and protein decomposition serve as nitrogen sources. Some bacteria are able to fix inorganic nitrogen (N_2).

Carbon—every organism must have a carbon source—autotrophic organisms can fix inorganic carbon (CO_2); heterotrophic organisms require an organic source of carbon (e.g., glucose).

Water—most metabolically active bacteria need a watery environment in which to live. If the salt concentration of the surrounding water is too high (i.e., is hypertonic), crenation of the cell may occur; however, some organisms (**halophiles**) require moderate to high salt concentrations.

Oxygen—microorganisms vary in their oxygen requirements. **Obligate aerobes** are those organisms that must have relatively large amounts of oxygen to grow. **Facultative anaerobes** can metabolize aerobically when oxygen is available, or anaerobically when it is not. Oxygen must be present for **microaerophiles** to grow, but only at low pressures (<0.2 atm O_2). Oxygen is toxic to **obligate anaerobes**, which cannot grow in the presence of oxygen. **Aerotolerant** organisms cannot metabolize aerobically, but are not harmed by the presence of oxygen.

CHAPTER 7

Control of Microbial Growth—Disinfection and Antisepsis

7.1 General Terms

There are various ways in which microbial growth can be retarded or inhibited. Some methods are as follows:

Sterilization—the process of killing (or removing) all microorganisms on an object or in a material (e.g., liquid media).

Disinfection—the process of reducing the numbers of or inhibiting the growth of microorganisms, especially pathogens, to the point where they no longer pose a threat of disease.

Disinfectant—a chemical agent used to destroy microorganisms on inanimate objects such as dishes, tables, and floors. Disinfectants are not safe for living tissues.

Antiseptic—a chemical agent that can be administered safely to external body surfaces or mucous membranes to decrease microbial numbers. Antiseptics cannot be taken internally.

-static agents—those that inhibit growth of microorganisms but do not kill them. A **bacteriostatic** agent is one that inhibits bacterial growth.

-cidal agents—those that kill microorganisms. A **bactericide** is a chemical agent that kills bacteria. A **viricide** is an agent that inactivates viruses. A **fungicide** is an agent that kills fungi. A **sporicide** is an agent that kills spores (bacterial or fungal).

Germicides—are broad-spectrum cidals, including both antiseptics and disinfectants.

Equivalent treatments—different methods or agents that produce the same results with regard to degree of antimicrobial capability.

Selective toxicity—term used to describe the activity of antimicrobial agents that are more harmful to the microbes than they are to the host—a desirable trait.

7.2 Factors Influencing Disinfectant Activity

Disinfectant activity is affected by the number of microorganisms, the species and types of microbes (some are more resistant than others, e.g., gram-positive bacteria are generally more sensitive to antibiotics than are gram-negative ones), physiology of organisms (growing organisms are more susceptible than dormant ones), environment (pH, presence or absence of organic matter), and temperature (increased temperatures generally enhance disinfectant activity).

Most antimicrobial agents exert their effect by damaging either the plasma membrane or proteins or nucleic acids.

7.3 Physical Methods

Heat is an economical and simple way to destroy microbes. All heat methods work by denaturing proteins.

Thermal death point (TDP)—the lowest temperature at which all bacteria in a liquid culture are killed within 10 minutes.

Thermal death time (TDT)—the time required to kill all bacteria in a liquid culture at a given temperature.

Decimal reduction time (DRT)—the time required to kill 90% of the bacteria in a liquid culture at a given temperature.

Moist heat methods include boiling, pasteurization, and autoclaving.

Boiling—very inexpensive and readily available; usually 100°C for 15 minutes—many vegetative cells and viruses are killed/inactivated within 10 minutes at 100°C.

Temperatures between 0° and 7°C may inhibit the reproduction of certain organisms or the production of toxins. However, these temperatures are rarely bactericidal. Freezing also may not be an effective method of disinfection. In fact, quick freezing is often used to store microorganisms for long periods of time. Slow freezing, however, causes severe damage to cellular constituents and may be bactericidal.

Pasteurization—primarily used to decrease the number of pathogenic organisms in food without adversely affecting the flavor; usually 72°C for 15 minutes or 63°C for 30 minutes.

Autoclaving—steam under pressure—the most effective moist heat method; usually 121.5°C at 15 psi for 15 minutes.

Dry heat methods of sterilization include direct flaming or incineration and hot air (160°C–170°C).

Desiccation—drying or freeze-drying can be used to inhibit growth (via inhibition of enzymes); organisms remain viable.

Osmotic pressure—extremely hypertonic conditions can cause plasmolysis (i.e., contraction of all the cell membrane away from the cell wall).

Filtration is a mechanical means of removing microorganisms. The liquid or gas is passed through a filter with pores small enough to prevent passage of microbes. This method can be used for substances that are sensitive to heat.

The effect of **radiation** is dependent on wavelength and on intensity and duration of exposure.

Ionizing radiation (alpha, beta, gamma, and x-rays, cathode rays, high-energy protons and neutrons) exhibits a high degree of penetrance. It creates free radicals in the medium, leading to the denaturation of proteins and nucleic acids. It can result in mutations. Viruses and spores are somewhat resistant.

Gram-negative bacteria are more sensitive to ionizing radiation than are gram-positive organisms.

Ultraviolet radiation is a form of nonionizing radiation. There is a low degree of penetration. It results in thymine dimers (cross-linkages) in DNA that interfere with replication.

Microwaves do not kill organisms directly, but they may be killed indirectly from heat generated in microwaved materials.

Visible light can cause oxidation of some light-sensitive materials.

7.4   Chemical Disinfection and Sterilization

Chemical methods are often referred to as **cold sterilization**. However, very few actually achieve sterilization.

The chemical structure of chlorhexidine is similar to hexachlorophene. **Chlorhexidine** is often combined with detergents or alcohol as a disinfectant of skin. It is an effective disinfectant of most vegetative bacteria and enveloped viruses. It is used in surgical hand scrubs.

Quaternary ammonium compounds or **quats** are cationic detergents. They are widely used. They are bactericidal against gram-positive bacteria, but less effective against gram-negative bacteria. Quats are also fungicidal, amoebicidal, and are effective against enveloped viruses. The mechanism of action of these detergents is unknown. However, the permeability of the membrane is probably affected, and they may also denature proteins.

7.5   Evaluating a Disinfectant

An ideal disinfectant quickly kills microorganisms without causing damage to the contaminated material. **Potency** is affected by concentration of the agent, length of exposure, temperature, and pH. Evaluation is difficult, but methods do exist, including the following:

Phenol coefficient test—compares the activity of a given agent relative to the killing power of phenol for the same amount of time under identical conditions.

Table 7.1 Chemical Disinfectants

Chemical Agent	Action	Examples
Phenolics	Very toxic, disrupt cell membranes and denature proteins	Phenol, cresol, hexachlorophene
Alcohols	Disrupt membranes and denature proteins	Ethanol, methanol, isopropanol
Aldehydes (alkylating agents)	Very effective, denature proteins	Formaldehyde, glutaraldehyde
Oxidizing agents	Very toxic to humans, oxidize molecules within cells, generate oxygen gas	Ozone, peroxide
Halogens	Negatively affected by presence of organic matter, oxidize cell components, disrupt membranes	Iodine, chlorine
Heavy metals	Inactivated by organic compounds, combine with sulfhydryl groups, denature proteins	Silver, mercury (very toxic), copper, zinc, selenium, arsenic
Surface-acting agents	Vary in degree, can simply reduce surface tension allowing organisms to be washed away, or may disrupt membranes and denature proteins	Soaps, detergents (including quaternary ammonium compounds), surfactants
Organic acids	Inhibit fungal metabolism (used as food preservatives)	Benzoic acid, propionic acid, sorbic acid
Gases	Denature proteins	Ethylene oxide (very toxic), vapors from formaldehyde, methyl bromide
Antiseptic dyes	Block cell wall synthesis, interfere with DNA replication	Acriflavine, crystal violet

Use-dilution test—rates agents by strength at various dilutions. A chemical that can be greatly diluted and still be effective gets a higher rating. A use-dilution is a dilution that kills all microorganisms at the 95% level of confidence.

Direct-spray method—used to test chemicals that are not water-soluble.

Tissue-toxicity test—tests antiseptics through exposure of tissue culture systems to dilutions of the agent.

7.6   Microbial Death

Bacteria that are treated with physical methods of microbial control or antimicrobial chemicals tend to die at a constant rate. When plotted on a semilogarithmic graph of log numbers of survivors versus time, the result is a straight line. Therefore, bacterial death is constant.

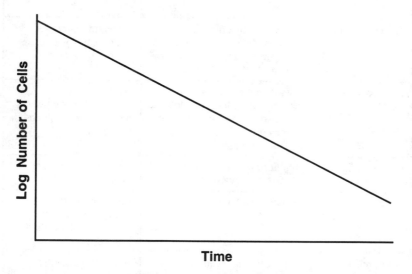

Figure 7.1 An Exponential Plot of the Surviving Cells Versus the Time of Exposure to a Lethal Agent

CHAPTER 8

Control of Microbial Growth—Antimicrobial Chemotherapy

8.1   General Terms

The ideal antimicrobial agent should be nontoxic to the host (selective toxicity), nonallergenic, soluble in body fluids, able to be maintained at therapeutic levels, have a low probability of eliciting resistance, long shelf life, and low cost.

Antibiotic—originally used to denote a chemical substance produced by one microorganism that kills or inhibits the growth of other microbes, the term now applies to both naturally produced substances and those synthesized in the laboratory. Most are produced by either fungi (e.g., penicillins, cephalosporins), *Bacillus* species (e.g., polymyxin, bacitracin), or *Streptomyces* species (streptomycin, tetracycline, erythromycin, kanamycin, neomycin, nystatin). Broad-spectrum antibiotics are those that act on both gram-positive and gram-negative bacteria.

Chemotherapeutic agent (drug)—any chemical (natural or synthetic) that is used in medicine. Ideally, it should attack microorganisms selectively and not harm human cells.

Natural drug—one made by microorganisms. **Synthetic drug**—one that is made in the laboratory. **Semisynthetic drug**—one synthesized partly in the laboratory and partly by microorganisms.

Synergistic effect—antibiotic effectiveness is often enhanced when given in combination with another drug. On the other hand, antagonistic effect is sometimes observed wherein certain combinations hinder antibiotic effectiveness.

Minimal inhibitory concentration (MIC)—the lowest drug concentration that will prevent growth of a standardized microbial suspension.

Minimal antibacterial (active) concentration (MAC)—the amount of drug (generally extremely small) that causes changes in cell morphology and inhibits growth.

8.2   Types of Agents

8.2.1   Antimycotics

Antimycotics (antifungals)—drugs that affect fungal growth, generally through inhibition of cell division, disruption of nucleic acid and protein synthesis, or changes in the cell membrane. Antifungal drugs include amphotericin B, clotrimazole, miconazole, and nystatin.

Polyene antibiotics are produced by a species of *Streptomyces* and are effective antifungal agents against opportunistic mycoses. These drugs combine with the sterols already present in the fungal membrane to change the permeability of the membrane. The result is cell death. These antibiotics are not effective against organisms that do not have sterols in their membranes and are therefore not bactericidal against them (mycoplasmas are the exception). **Nystatin** is used against *Candida* infections.

Clotrimazole and **miconazole** are **imidazole antifungals**, which may be used against cutaneous mycoses such as athlete's foot. **Ketoconazole** is an imidazole antifungal, which is used against systemic mycoses. These imidazole antifungals interfere with sterol synthesis and inhibit the formation of a fully functional fungal membrane.

Triazole antifungals include **fluconazole** and **itraconazole**. Both are used for systemic mycoses.

Griseofulvin is produced by a *Penicillium* and interferes with mitosis. It is effective when taken orally against superficial dermatophytic mycoses of the hair. It acts by disrupting cell division.

8.2.2 Antiprotozoals

Antiprotozoals—drugs that affect the growth of protozoans; often toxic and not always easy to obtain. Examples include **quinacrine hydrochloride** and **metronidazole**.

8.2.3 Antivirals

Antiviral agents must be shown to be nontoxic to humans before they can be used. The **interferons** (IFNs) are a group of antiviral and antitumor proteins. They are released from virus-infected cells, causing neighboring cells to make antiviral proteins. Interferons inhibit viral replication. Recombinant DNA technology is used to produce high levels of interferons. The three types are alpha, beta, and gamma IFNs. Other antiviral agents include **acyclovir**, **amantadine**, and **5-iodo-2′-deoxyuridine**.

8.2.4 Antihelminthics

Niclosamide is an **antihelminthic drug** used against the beef tapeworm *(Taenia saginata)*. **Praziquantel** is used against tapeworms as well as some flukes, including *Schistosomas*. **Mebendazole** is used against *Ascaris lumbricoids, Enterobius vermicularis*, and *Trichuris trichiura*. **Piperazine** is used to paralyze pinworms and ascariasis.

8.3 Mechanisms of Action of Antimicrobial Drugs

Cidal drugs cause irreversible damage or death and are independent of host activity. **Static drugs** inhibit growth or reproduction and are dependent on the immune system of the host for elimination of pathogens from the body.

Antimicrobial agents can inhibit growth or kill microbes through inhibition of nucleic acid synthesis, protein synthesis, cell wall formation, or metabolic products or by damaging the plasma membrane, causing cell lysis.

8.3.1   Cell Wall Synthesis

Peptidoglycan is unique to bacterial cell walls. Antibiotics that prevent the synthesis of peptidoglycans weaken the cell wall of the bacteria and cause cell lysis. Penicillin prevents the synthesis of peptidoglycans and is effective against gram-positive bacteria. The lipopolysaccharides of the outer membrane of gram-negative bacteria allow these bacteria to be resistant to these types of antibiotics. Bacitracin, vancomycin, cephalosporins, and penicillin are antibiotics that interfere with the synthesis of peptidoglycans. These antibiotics do not affect the eukaryotic host cells because eukaryotic cells do not contain peptidoglycans.

8.3.2   Protein Synthesis

Chloramphenicol, erythromycin, streptomycin, and tetracyclines are antibiotics that interfere with **protein synthesis**. These antibiotics interfere with the bacterial ribosomes involved in the process of synthesizing a protein strand. These antibiotics do not affect the eukaryotic cells because eukaryotes use different ribosomes in protein synthesis.

8.3.3   Plasma Membranes

Disruption of the cell membrane causes a change in the permeability of the cell and can cause cell lysis. Polymyxin B attaches to the phospholipids of the membranes. Nystatin, amphotericin B, miconazole, and ketoconazole are effective antifungals that selectively cause the increased permeability of the fungal membrane because these attach to the sterols in the fungal membrane. Animal cells also contain sterols; therefore, some of these drugs may be toxic to the host.

8.3.4   Replication

Idoxuridine, rifamycin, and quinolones are antibiotics that interfere with **DNA replication** and **transcription**. However, these may also interfere with host replication and transcription. Selective toxicity is vital in the effectiveness of the antibiotic.

8.3.5   Synthesis of Essential Metabolites

Antibiotics that compete with microbial enzymes may be effective chemotherapies. Sulfonamides and dapsone inhibit the synthesis of folic acid in many microorganisms. The inhibition of folic acid synthesis causes the microorganism to stop growing. Humans do not produce folic acid by this metabolic pathway. Human host cells are therefore not affected by these drugs. Trimethoprim blocks tetrahydrofolate synthesis, and isoniazid is thought to inhibit the synthesis of mycolic acid.

8.4 Evaluating an Antimicrobial Drug

There are a number of methods for testing the sensitivity of microbes to antibiotics; these include **serum killing power, Kirby-Bauer disk diffusion,** and automated techniques.

Serum killing power—tests activity of the antibiotic in the patient's serum. The patient's serum is drawn during the time period when the patient is receiving the antibiotic. A bacterial suspension is added to the serum to see if the microbes are affected.

Disk diffusion method (Kirby-Bauer)—infecting microorganisms are cultured on agar plates and subjected to filter disks that have been impregnated with various antibiotics. Cleared **zones of inhibition** indicate antibiotic sensitivity.

8.5 Side Effects

Drugs vary in effectiveness and in the number and degree of severity of **side effects**. Side effects of antimicrobial agents include toxicity, allergic response, and disruption of normal flora.

Many drugs attack not only the infectious organisms, but the normal flora as well. **Superinfections** with new pathogens can occur when the defensive capacity of the host's normal flora is compromised or destroyed.

8.6 Drug Resistance

Resistance to an antibiotic means that a microorganism that was formerly susceptible to the action of that antibiotic is no longer affected by it. Antibiotic resistance can sometimes be transferred among bacteria on extrachromosomal DNA molecules known as plasmids. Resistance may be due to changes in the sensitivity of affected enzymes, changes in the selective permeability of cell walls and membranes, increased production of a competitive substrate, or enzymatic alteration of the drug itself.

Unnecessary exposure to antibiotics has brought about a significant increase in **antibiotic-resistant microbes**. This calls into question the routine uses of antibiotics such as feed additives for livestock and food additives used to prolong freshness in agricultural products. These practices create conditions that are conducive to the development of resistant strains that may be transferred to a human host when the product is ingested.

Nosocomial infections are infections acquired during a hospital stay. They are often extremely resistant to antibiotics and very difficult to treat.

A group of gram-negative bacteria are resistant to disinfectants and antiseptics; they are the **Pseudomonads** (genus *Pseudomonas*). Pseudomonads may even thrive and grow in the presence of disinfectants and antiseptics. The resistance of these bacteria is thought to be due to the presence of **porins** in the membrane. Porins are proteins that form channels, which permit small molecules to flow into and out of the cell.

Mycobacterium tuberculosis, the causative agent in **tuberculosis**, is also resistant to disinfectants, as well as antibiotics.

Endospores and cysts of bacteria and protozoa, respectively, are also resistant to disinfectants.

8.7 Some Common Antibacterial Drugs

Penicillins (including ampicillins and cephalosporins)—narrow-spectrum bactericides; interfere with cell wall formation; effective only against vegetative cells of gram-positive sensitive species. Susceptible to beta-lactamase activity.

Some organisms, such as *Haemophilus influenzae, Neisseria gonorrhoeae*, and *Staphylococcus aureus*, produce an enzyme known as beta-lactamase. The presence of this enzyme makes the organisms resistant to beta-lactam antibiotics—namely, penicillins and cephalosporins.

Monobactams—effective against aerobic, gram-negative organisms (e.g., *Enterobacter, Haemophilus, Neisseria*); stable to beta-lactamase.

Chloramphenicol and **tetracyclines**—broad-spectrum bacteriostatics that act on both gram-positive and gram-negative bacteria; inhibit protein synthesis.

Aminoglycosides (including kanamycin and streptomycin)—bactericidal; interfere with protein synthesis.

Polymyxin B and **colistin**—disrupt the plasma membrane, allowing cytoplasmic constituents to leak out.

Sulfa drugs—bacteriostatic; active upon vegetative cells; competitively inhibit enzymes.

CHAPTER 9

Microbial Genetics

9.1   Genetics

Genetics is the study of genes, what they are, and how they work, including how they store, express, and replicate information, and how that information is transmitted to subsequent generations (**heredity**). A **gene** is a segment of DNA, composed of a sequence of nucleotides that specify the structure of a functional product, usually a protein.

DNA—deoxyribonucleic acid, the genetic substance of a cell. DNA exists as a double-stranded, helical molecule (see figure 9.1). The two strands are composed of a series of nitrogenous bases (A = adenine, T = thymine, G = guanine, and C = cytosine) that are connected by sugar-phosphate molecules. The nitrogenous bases opposing each other along the two strands are linked by hydrogen bonds (adenine pairs with thymine; guanine with cytosine). Each base pair is composed of one purine (A or G) and one pyrimidine (T or C).

9.2   Chromosomes

A **chromosome** is a single DNA molecule, composed of one long double helix and containing all or a part of the genome. Eukaryotic chromosomes have proteins known as **histones** associated with them; these proteins regulate gene

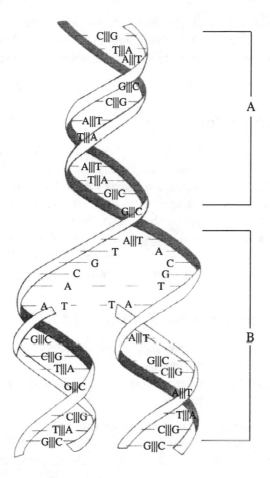

Figure 9.1 DNA. The double helix (A) is found in an undividing eukaryotic cell. The lower section (B) has been uncoiled, and each template strand is being replicated.

activity. Prokaryotic chromosomes do not have these associated proteins and are said to be **naked**.

Prokaryotes have a single, circular chromosome. Asexual reproduction leads to two daughter cells—each receiving a chromosome that is identical to the original parental chromosome.

Plasmids are circular, extrachromosomal DNA molecules that are generally not essential for cell survival.

Eukaryotes have multiple, linear chromosomes. Reproduction may be asexual, with each new cell receiving chromosomes identical to the parent cell, or sexual, in which the new cell receives a subset of genetic information from each parent.

9.3   Replication

For DNA replication to occur, the two strands of the double helix must separate. The point where they are separated is called the **replication fork**. Each separated strand serves as a **template** for **DNA polymerases** in the synthesis of a new strand. Because of the rules of nitrogenous base pairing (i.e., A pairs only with T, and G pairs only with C), the sequence along the old strand dictates precisely the sequence along the new strand. Each new double-stranded DNA molecule contains one old strand and one new strand; thus, the process of DNA replication is said to be **semiconservative.**

9.4   Transcription—Synthesis of RNA

Transcription is the synthesis of single-stranded RNA (ribonucleic acid) molecules based on a DNA sequence. The two strands of the DNA must pull apart temporarily, allowing **RNA polymerase** to access the DNA for use as a template for RNA production.

RNA is synthesized from adenine (A), guanine (G), cytosine (C), and uracil (U). Thymine is not present in RNA. The As, Gs, Cs, and Ts along the DNA template produce Us, Cs, Gs, and As, respectively, along the RNA strand being synthesized.

Three kinds of RNA may be produced: (1) **ribosomal RNA (rRNA)**, which combines with proteins to form ribosomes (where new proteins are synthesized), (2) **transfer RNA (tRNA)**, which transports amino acids to the ribosome for assembly into proteins, and (3) **messenger RNA (mRNA)**, which dictates the sequence of amino acid assembly.

Transcription occurs in the cytoplasm of prokaryotes, while it occurs in the nucleus of eukaryotes.

Eukaryotic mRNA contains regions that are not used for protein synthesis (the **introns**), as well as those regions that are (the **exons**). Prior to mRNA transport out of the nucleus, enzymes remove the introns, and the **spliceosome** connects the exons into a functional mRNA that is then exported to the cytoplasm.

9.5 Translation

Translation is the process wherein information in the form of nitrogenous bases along an mRNA is translated into the amino acid sequence of a protein.

The sequence of nucleotides along the mRNA is "read" in groups of three; each group of three is called a **triplet** or **codon**. Codons in mRNA pair with anticodons found in tRNA molecules. The triplet **anticodon** is located at one point on the tRNA molecule while the corresponding amino acid is attached to the tRNA at another point. The mRNA and tRNA are brought together at the ribosome. The ribosome moves along the mRNA strand during the synthesis of the polypeptide.

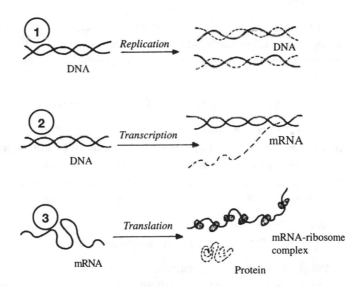

Figure 9.2 Summary: Replication, Transcription, and Translation. (1) This DNA is used in the nucleus of new cells. (2) The mRNA leaves the nucleus and is used in protein synthesis. (3) Amino acids are assembled onto the mRNA-ribosome complex to create a protein.

The mRNA codons make up the **genetic code**, which is essentially identical among all living things. The code comprises 64 codons—61 code for amino acids (these are the **sense codons**), while 3 do not code for amino acids but function as stop signals for the translation process (these are the **nonsense codons**). There are 61 codons coding for 21 amino acids; thus, some amino acids are coded for by more than one codon. Hence, the code is said to be **degenerate**. The **start codon** is AUG and codes for the amino acid methionine.

A **polypeptide** is a chain of amino acids.

A **polyribosome** is an mRNA with many ribosomes attached.

Due to the absence of a nuclear membrane, prokaryotic translation can begin even before transcription is completed. This is not so in eukaryotic cells, in which transcription occurs in the nucleus and translation occurs in the cytoplasm.

9.6 Mutation

Mutations—changes in the sequence of A, T, G, and C along a DNA strand. Mutations are changes in the genotype; they may or may not change the phenotype (the observable characteristics). A **silent mutation** does not alter the phenotype.

Mutations may be **neutral, harmful,** or **beneficial** in their effect.

Spontaneous mutations—occur naturally, appear to be due to random errors in base pairing during DNA replication. **Induced mutations** occur as a result of exposure to a **mutagen**—a chemical substance or physical factor that increases the mutation rate; it causes permanent damage to the DNA. Examples include ultraviolet light, nitrous oxide, and benzo(a)pyrene.

Mutation rate—the probability that a mutation will occur in a gene when the cell divides. Different genes have different mutation rates.

Point mutation (base substitution)—change in a single nucleotide; may result in no change in amino acid (**silent mutation**), substitution of a different amino acid (**missense mutation**), or creation of a stop codon (**nonsense mutation**).

Frameshift mutation—a base pair is inserted or deleted; this generally affects the mRNA from that point on, i.e., it can change all triplets for the rest of the sequence. The changes may include silent, missense, and nonsense mutations. Frameshift mutations are more likely to result in a deficient protein product than are point mutations.

9.6.1 Detecting Mutants

Mutants can be identified by **selecting** or testing for an altered phenotype.

Positive selection—mutant cells are selected and nonmutant cells are inhibited.

Negative selection—the **replica plating** technique is used to identify mutants that cannot grow under the selective conditions.

An **auxotroph** is a mutant with a nutritional requirement that was not present in the parent. For example, a histidine auxotroph is a bacterium that cannot grow unless histidine is added to the medium.

9.6.2 Mutagens

The following are examples of **chemical mutagens: base analogs** such as 2-aminopurine, which incorporates in place of thymine; **base-pair mutagens** such as nitrous acid, which converts adenine into hypoxanthine; and frameshift mutagens such as benzo(a)pyrene. Others include alkylating agents, deaminating agents, and acridine derivatives.

Ionizing and ultraviolet radiation are also mutagens. Ionizing radiation can cause base substitutions, disrupt the sugar-phosphate backbone, or create reactive free radicals. Ultraviolet radiation causes thymine dimers, i.e., bonding between adjacent thymines.

9.6.3 Repair of DNA Damage

Some bacteria have enzymes that can repair DNA. There are two kinds of repair: **light repair**, in which a light-activated enzyme breaks thymine-thymine bonds; and **dark repair**, in which several different enzymes are involved in excising defective DNA and resynthesizing the DNA strand based on the nonmutated strand.

9.6.4   Identifying Carcinogens

The **Ames test** for the identification of carcinogens is based on the assumptions that (1) the presence of a mutagen can cause mutant cells to revert back to their original state, and (2) many mutagens are also carcinogens. The test involves exposure of histidine auxotrophs of *Salmonella* to a suspected mutagen, followed by selection for nonmutant cells. The presence of nonmutant *Salmonella* indicates a positive test for mutagenicity. The Ames test is quick and relatively inexpensive.

9.7   Gene Transfer

Gene transfer—the movement of genetic information from one bacterium to another. There are three processes for genetic transfer in bacteria: **transformation, transduction,** and **conjugation.** All of these are significant in that they bring about an increase in the amount of genetic variation within a population.

9.7.1   Transformation

Transformation—"naked" DNA is transferred from one bacterium to another in solution. DNA fragments are released as double-stranded DNA into the medium. **Endonucleases** cut the double-stranded DNA in solution and the resulting fragments separate—only single-stranded molecules are transferred. The transferred DNA is spliced into the recipient cell's DNA. Uptake is dependent upon the presence of a protein known as competence factor. **Bacterial competence** is the ability of a bacterium to take up DNA from the extracellular environment.

Transformation occurs naturally among some bacteria. It is used in the laboratory to create recombinant DNA and is also used to study the effects of introducing DNA into a cell, and in mapping gene locations.

9.7.1.1   The Experiments of Griffith and Avery

The following experiment of Frederick Griffith (1928) demonstrated transformation. There are two kinds of pneumococcus cells—rough and smooth. Only the smooth form is **virulent** (i.e., capable of infecting and killing mice). Griffith showed that neither heat-killed smooth cells nor live rough cells alone

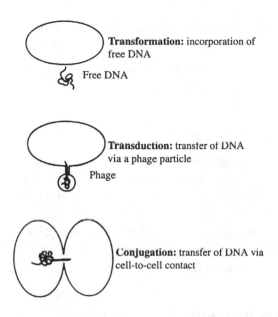

Transformation: incorporation of free DNA

Free DNA

Transduction: transfer of DNA via a phage particle

Phage

Conjugation: transfer of DNA via cell-to-cell contact

Figure 9.3 Summary: Three Methods of Gene Transfer in Bacteria

were capable of causing infection. However, when live rough cells were mixed with heat-killed smooth cells, the mice died and live smooth cells could be recovered. Oswald T. Avery (1940) showed that only the smooth cells contained the capsular polysaccharide that is responsible for virulence, and that the substance involved in the transfer was neither a protein nor the polysaccharide itself. Instead, it was the DNA containing the gene for the capsular polysaccharide that was being transferred from the dead smooth cells to the live rough cells, transforming them into the virulent smooth pneumococci.

9.7.2 Transduction

Transduction—DNA is transferred from one bacterium to another via a bacteriophage and then incorporated into the recipient's DNA. The bacterial virus may be virulent or temperate (i.e., a prophage).

9.7.3 Conjugation

Conjugation—DNA is transferred from one live bacterium to another through direct contact; large quantities of DNA can be transferred in this way.

F factors—plasmids transferred from a donor cell (an F⁺ cell) to a recipient cell (an F⁻ cell) during conjugation.

An **Hfr (high frequency of recombination)** is a cell with an F plasmid incorporated into the chromosome.

9.8 Recombination

Genetic recombination—rearrangement of genes from separate groups of genes. Genes from two chromosomes are recombined into one chromosome containing some genes from each of the original chromosomes. This contributes to genetic diversity. In eukaryotes, the process is associated with sexual reproduction, during which haploid gametes, produced by meiosis, fuse to form a diploid zygote. Portions of chromosomes may be exchanged during meiosis by a process known as crossing-over.

9.9 Transposons

Transposons—small DNA segments that can move from one part of a chromosome to another area on either the same chromosome, a different chromosome, or a plasmid. They may be **simple** or **complex**. A simple transposon, or insertion sequence, is a short segment of DNA that contains only those genes coding for the enzymes responsible for its transposition. Complex transposons can carry any type of gene, including those for antibiotic resistance, and are an important natural mechanism for gene movement.

9.10 Recombinant DNA Technology

Genetic engineering—manipulated gene transfer in the laboratory.

Recombinant DNA—DNA that has been artificially altered to combine genes from different sources.

Biotechnology—application of genetic engineering and use of recombinant DNA in research, medicine, industry, and agriculture (see also Chapter 12).

Vector—piece of DNA used to transfer DNA between organisms. The gene of interest is inserted into the vector (usually a plasmid or a viral genome), which is then transferred into a new cell. The new cell is used to grow a **clone** from which large amounts of the gene or its product can be harvested. Some vectors contain antibiotic-resistance genes, or **markers**, that can be used to identify cells containing the vector.

Restriction enzyme—an enzyme that recognizes and cuts a specific DNA sequence. They are generally named for the microorganism in which they were first discovered; e.g., the restriction enzyme *EcoRI* was isolated from *Escherichia coli;* it recognizes and cuts the sequence GAATTC.

Gene library—an entire genome cut with restriction enzymes and inserted into vector molecules.

cDNA—DNA synthesized from a strand of mRNA by reverse transcription; the required enzyme is **reverse transcriptase**, which was originally isolated from a retrovirus.

Clone identification can be accomplished through replica plating.

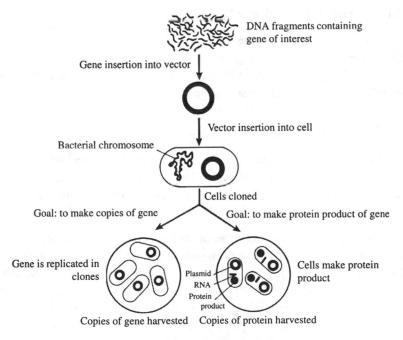

Figure 9.4 Genetic Engineering

9.11 Diversity and Evolution

Mutation, gene transfer, and recombination are all important in increasing genetic diversity. **Diversity** is a necessary prerequisite for evolution.

9.12 Regulation of Gene Expression in Bacteria

Constitutive enzymes—those that are always present. **Constitutive genes** are those that continue to produce proteins regardless of other factors, including the concentrations of substrate and end product. For example, most glycolytic enzymes (and the genes that produce them) are constitutive.

Other enzymes are regulated at the genetic level and are described as **inducible**. Regulatory mechanisms such as **induction, repression,** and **attenuation** are ways to control the activity of genes to determine which mRNAs are synthesized and, therefore, which proteins will be made.

9.12.1 The Operon Model

An **operon** consists of three segments: a promoter, an operator, and structural genes. When the repressor, which is the protein that binds to the operator, is removed, transcription can take place. Gene expression occurs once transcription of the structural genes is set in motion.

9.12.2 Enzyme Induction

In the **operon model for an inducible system**, the presence of an inducer activates an operon and the cell synthesizes more enzymes. In some cases, the inducer binds to the repressor so that it cannot bind to the operator and prevent transcription.

Beta-galactosidase and the lac operon is an example of an inducible system. Beta-galactosidase is an enzyme involved in the metabolism of lactose. Lactose is the inducer for the operon controlling production of beta-galactosidase. When lactose is absent, a repressor is produced that binds to the operator and inactivates the operon—beta-galactosidase is not produced. When lactose is present, it inactivates the repressor, thus allowing transcription to occur and beta-galactosidase is produced.

9.12.3 Enzyme Repression

In the **operon model for a repressible system,** a repressor binds to the operator and prevents transcription; in some cases the repressor cannot bind to the operator site without a **corepressor,** and it is the presence or absence of the corepressor that controls synthesis.

The repressor is often a synthetic product that inhibits further production of the enzyme responsible for its synthesis. **Tryptophan and the trp operon** illustrate enzyme repression. When tryptophan is present, it attaches to and activates a regulator protein that represses the trp operon. When tryptophan is not present, the repressor is not activated and transcription of the trp operon can occur.

Catabolite repression—the presence of glucose (or some other preferred nutrient) represses synthesis of the enzymes necessary to metabolize an alternative substance.

9.12.4 Attenuation

Attenuation is a form of regulation wherein mRNA synthesis is prematurely terminated at a point called the **attenuator** site.

CHAPTER 10

Role of Microbes in Disease

10.1   Host–Microbe Relationships

An organism that harbors another organism is called a **host**.

Normal (indigenous) flora—those microorganisms that can establish populations in a host, such as the human body, without causing disease. These microorganisms are called normal (indigenous) flora.

Opportunistic flora are those microorganisms that do not normally cause disease but may do so under certain conditions (e.g., when the host is immunocompromised); they may be resident or transient.

Resident flora are those with permanent populations.

Transient flora are those with temporary or semipermanent populations.

Microbial antagonism is a phenomenon wherein the normal flora prevent pathogens from causing infection.

10.1.1   Symbiosis: Commensalism, Mutualism, and Parasitism

A relationship wherein two organisms live together is called a **symbiosis**; there are three types:

Commensalism—one of the two organisms benefits from the relationship, the other is unaffected.

Mutualism—both organisms benefit from the relationship.

Parasitism—one organism benefits and the other is harmed.

10.1.2 Pathogens

Pathogen—a parasitic microorganism that causes disease.

Pathogenicity—the ability of a microbe to produce disease.

Virulence—the power of an organism to cause disease.

Infection—pathogen invasion of the body.

Disease—disturbed health due to a pathogen or other factor.

Pathogens gain access to a host via a portal of entry and leave via a portal of exit.

Portals of entry include the mucous membranes (including those lining the respiratory, gastrointestinal, and genitourinary tracts) and parenteral entry (direct inoculation through the skin via bites, injections, or other wounds). The most frequently used portal of entry is the respiratory tract. Many pathogens cannot cause infection unless they enter through a specific (**preferred**) portal of entry.

Portals of exit include the respiratory tract (through coughing and sneezing), the gastrointestinal tract (through saliva and feces), and secretions from the genitourinary tract. Microbes may also leave the body via blood into syringes or biting arthropods.

10.2 Kinds of Disease

An **infectious disease** is one caused by an organism that can be transmitted.

A **communicable (contagious) disease** can be spread from one organism (host) to another. A noncommunicable disease cannot be spread in this way and is usually contracted from an environmental source, such as soil or water.

A **primary infection** occurs in a previously noninfected individual.

Secondary infections are those that occur once a host is weakened from a **primary** infection.

A **systemic infection** is spread throughout the body, while a **local infection** is limited to a small area of the body.

An **endogenous disease** is one caused by a pathogen, usually an opportunistic organism, from within the body, while an **exogenous disease** is one caused by a pathogen or other factors from outside the body.

A **chronic disease** is one in which symptoms are slow to develop and the disease is slow to disappear. An **acute disease** progresses quickly.

Latent symptoms appear (or reappear) long after infection.

An infection that does not cause any signs of disease is said to be **inapparent** or **subclinical**.

A **mixed infection** is one caused by two or more pathogens.

Syndrome—a characteristic group of signs and symptoms that always accompanies a specific disease.

10.3 How Microbes Cause Disease

Bacterial pathogens must first adhere to a host. **Adhesins** are projections on the surface of the bacterium that adhere to complementary receptors on host cells. **Adherence** is followed by **colonization** of the tissues (in complex multicellular organisms), and may also involve **invasion** of cells.

Disease-causing bacteria may produce toxins or special enzymes. **Hemolysins**, which destroy red blood cells, and **leukocidins**, which destroy neutrophils and macrophages, are both special enzymes produced by pathogenic bacteria. Other such enzymes include **coagulase**, which helps in blood clotting; **fibrinolysin**, which breaks down blood clots; and **hyaluronidase**, which destroys a mucopolysaccharide that holds cells together in tissues.

Staphylokinase is produced by *Staphylococcus aureus*. **Bacterial kinases** are used to dissolve clots in plasma, which is the host cell's attempt to isolate the infection.

Collagenase is produced by *Clostridium* (spp) and breaks down the connective tissue of the host, allowing the pathogen to spread.

M protein is produced by *Streptococcus pyogenes* and assists the attachment of the bacterium to the host epithelial lining. The M protein increases the virulence of the bacterium.

The **capsule** is an indication of the virulence of the microorganism. It increases the virulence by inhibiting the host's natural defense of phagocytosis.

Necrotizing factors are produced by bacteria and cause the death of somatic cells. Necrotizing factors increase the virulence of the bacterium.

10.3.1 Bacterial Toxins

Bacterial toxins include exotoxins and endotoxins.

10.3.1.1 Exotoxins

Exotoxins are produced and excreted mostly by gram-positive bacteria into the surroundings as the pathogen grows. Exotoxins are proteins that usually have enzymatic activity. There are three types of exotoxins: **cytotoxins**, which cause the death of host cells; **neurotoxins**, which interfere with the normal nervous function; and **enterotoxins**, which affect the intestinal lining of the host.

The host immune system produces **antitoxins** in the form of antibodies against bacterial exotoxins. Exotoxins may also be inactivated by heat or chemical treatment. **Toxoids** are altered exotoxins that allow the host immune system to produce antitoxins without causing any side effects. Toxoids may be used as vaccines against the microorganisms that produce the exotoxins.

Corynebacterium diphtheriae produces **diphtheria toxin,** which is cytotoxic to human cells by causing inhibition of protein synthesis. This toxin contains two polypeptides, one that causes symptoms and one that causes binding of the bacterium to the host cell. Diphtheria can be prevented by using a toxoid as a vaccine.

Streptococcus pyogenes produces three cytotoxic **erythrogenic exotoxins,** which cause the characteristic skin rash in scarlet fever.

Clostridium botulinum produces the neurotoxin **botulinum toxin**. Botulinum toxin binds to acetylcholine, a neurotransmitter, and causes paralysis.

Clostridium tetani produces the neurotoxin **tetanospasmin** or the **tetanus toxin**. This toxin binds specifically to cells that control the contraction of skeletal muscle. The result of toxin binding is uncontrollable muscle contraction (lockjaw).

Vibrio cholerae produces the enterotoxin cholera toxin. The **vibrio enterotoxin** consists of two polypeptides, one involved in the symptoms of the disease and the second involved in binding. The bacteria bind to the host's intestinal epithelium and cause the epithelium to excrete fluids and electrolytes. The result is diarrhea, vomiting, and disturbances of normal muscular contraction.

Staphylococcus aureus produces a **staphylococcal enterotoxin** that causes toxic shock syndrome.

10.3.2   Endotoxins

Endotoxins are produced by gram-negative bacteria and are located in the outer membrane of the bacteria. The lipid component of the **lipopolysaccharides (LPS)** is the endotoxin. Endotoxins are not secreted by the bacterial cells. The bacterial cell must die and the outer membrane be broken down for the endotoxin to be released into the bloodstream. The host's responses to endotoxins include chills, fever, weakness, generalized aches, and, in severe cases, shock and death.

The host macrophage in response to the phagocytosis of the gram-negative bacteria secrete **interleukin-1 (IL-1)**. IL-1 causes the hypothalamus to release prostaglandins and results in fever.

Severe reactions to endotoxins include septic or endotoxic shock. Phagocytosis of the gram-negative bacteria causes the secretion of **tumor necrosis factor (TNF)** or **cachectin** from host phagocytes. The net effect of the secretion of these are increases in tissue fluid loss, loss of blood pressure, and shock.

Pathogenic viruses, fungi, protozoans, and helminths also damage host cells and tissues.

Cytopathic effects (CPEs) are the signs of cell damage due to viral infection.

Viruses also release digestive enzymes and alter host DNA.

Fungal pathogens digest cells; some produce toxins or allergic reactions.

Protozoans and helminths produce symptoms through direct damage to host tissues, release of toxic waste products, or by causing allergic reactions.

10.4 The Disease Process

Signs of disease are objective changes that can be observed and measured.

Symptoms are subjective changes reported by the patient.

Physicians use both signs and symptoms in making a **diagnosis** (identification of a disease).

Incubation period—the time interval between infection and the appearance of signs and symptoms.

Prodromal period—pathogens are beginning to invade host tissues; characterized by the appearance of early signs and symptoms that are generally nonspecific in nature.

Period of illness—disease is at its most severe; all signs and symptoms are present and at their worst. This is also known as the **invasive** phase. The term **acme**, or **critical**, stage is used to describe the period of most intense symptoms.

Period of decline—signs and symptoms begin to subside; host defenses overcome the pathogens.

Period of convalescence—tissue damage is repaired and the body returns to its healthy, prediseased state.

10.5 Koch's Postulates

Koch's postulates provide a method for demonstrating that a specific microorganism transmits a specific disease.

Koch's postulates are as follows:

1. The microorganism must be obtained from a diseased animal (the microbe must be found in every animal that has the disease).

2. The microbe is isolated and grown in pure culture.

3. The cultured organism is inoculated into a healthy animal, which then contracts the same disease.

4. Identical microorganisms are recovered from the diseased animal and re-isolated in pure culture.

10.5.1 Exceptions to Koch's Postulates

Some microbial pathogens cause more than one disease, e.g., *Streptococcus pyogenes.*

Some diseases may be caused by more than one microbial pathogen, e.g., pneumonia.

Some diseases do not always exhibit the same signs and symptoms, e.g., tetanus.

Some pathogens cannot be grown on artificial media.

10.6 Epidemiology

Epidemiology is the study of the factors and mechanisms involved in the spread of infectious disease; it deals with transmission, incidence, prevalence, and frequency of disease.

Transmission—how a disease is spread among hosts.

Incidence—the number of *new* cases of a disease over a specific period of time.

Prevalence—the number of cases of a disease at a given point in time.

Morbidity rate—the number of cases of the disease, expressed as a proportion of the population.

Mortality rate—the number of deaths attributed to the disease, expressed as a proportion of the population.

Frequency of occurrence may be described as sporadic, endemic, epidemic, or pandemic.

Sporadic—a few isolated cases exist in the population.

Endemic—a large number of cases exist, but do not appear to pose a significant health threat.

Epidemic—a large number of cases exist and are causing patients sufficient harm so as to constitute a significant threat to public health. Epidemics may stem from a **common source** of infection, such as a water supply, or they may be **propagated** through person-to-person contact.

Pandemic—an epidemic disease occurring over an exceptionally large geographic area or areas.

Data on the incidence and prevalence of **reportable** infectious diseases are reported to public health officials on local, state, federal, and world levels. The Centers for Disease Control (CDC), the main source of epidemiological information in the United States, publishes such information in its *Morbidity and Mortality Weekly Report* (MMWR).

10.6.1 Reservoirs

A **reservoir** is a living or nonliving source from which an infectious disease can be spread. Living sources include people who have the disease or are carriers of the disease. Soil, water, and waste materials are all examples of nonliving reservoirs of infection.

Zoonoses are diseases that are transmitted from an animal reservoir to humans. Transmission may be by direct contact or through a vector.

10.6.2 Transmission

Disease may be transmitted through **direct** or **indirect** contact with a reservoir of infection, or through a vector.

There are two kinds of **direct contact** transmission—**vertical transmission**, i.e., parent to child, and **horizontal transmission**, i.e., person-to-person transmissions other than parent to child.

Indirect contact may occur through **droplets** of saliva or mucus, or through contact with **fomites** (inanimate objects that are contaminated with infectious organisms).

Transmission through a medium such as air, water, or food is known as **vehicle transmission**.

Arthropod vectors (e.g., ticks, fleas, mosquitoes) can transmit pathogens from one host to another by both biological and mechanical means.

Epidemic control measures include elimination of the reservoir, elimination of the vector, immunization of susceptible individuals, and quarantine of infected individuals.

10.7 Host Defense Mechanisms

Resistance—the ability to ward off disease. It is the result of genetically predetermined (**innate**) resistance and other factors such as the individual's age, sex, and nutritional status. **Susceptibility** is lack of resistance.

Predisposing factors, such as age, fatigue, stress, and poor nutrition, can make a host more susceptible to infection and disease.

Nonspecific defenses (e.g., fever, inflammation) are used to protect the body from all kinds of pathogenic organisms. They generally serve as a first line of defense.

Specific defenses include **innate resistance** and **acquired resistance** to specific pathogens (**immunity**). Types of immunity will be discussed further in section 10.7.2.

10.7.1 Nonspecific Host Defense Mechanisms

Nonspecific defenses include **mechanical barriers** such as skin, saliva, the lacrimal apparatus, and mucous membranes, as well as the outward flow of urine, vaginal secretions, and blood (from wounds). **Phagocytosis, fever, inflammation**, and **molecular strategies** are discussed below.

There are three categories of white blood cells (**leukocytes**): the **granulocytes** (neutrophils, basophils, eosinophils), which predominate early in infection; the **monocytes**, which predominate late in infection; and the **lymphocytes.**

Phagocytosis is the cellular ingestion of a foreign substance (including microorganisms). Certain types of white blood cells (including neutrophils and monocytes in the blood, and fixed and wandering macrophages) are **phagocytes.**

Phagocytes locate microorganisms through chemotaxis. They then adhere to the microbial cells, a process that is sometimes facilitated by **opsonization,** wherein the microbial cell is coated with plasma proteins. Pseudopods then encircle and engulf the microbe. The phagocytized microbe, enclosed in a vacuole called a **phagosome**, is usually killed by lysosomal enzymes and oxidizing agents.

Fever is abnormally high body temperature produced in response to infection. It serves to augment the immune system, inhibit microbial growth, increase the rate of chemical reactions, raise the temperature above the organism's optimum growth temperature, and decrease patient activity.

Inflammation is a response to cell damage. Initiation of inflammation is caused by the release of histamine, kinins, and prostaglandins. Redness, heat, swelling, pain, and sometimes loss of function are characteristic of inflammation.

Tissue injury also stimulates **blood clotting**, which may help to prevent dissemination of the infection.

Interferons (see Section 8.2.3) are produced in response to viral infections. They cause uninfected cells to produce **antiviral proteins** (AVPs).

The **complement system** refers to a group of blood serum proteins that activate a **cascade** series of reactions to destroy invading pathogens. It causes cell lysis, inflammation, and opsonization. Complement deficiencies result in reduced resistance to infection.

10.7.2 Specific Host Defense Mechanisms—Types of Immunity

Immunity—the ability of the body to recognize and defend itself against an infectious agent.

Specific immunity is characterized by specificity, recognition of self vs. nonself, heterogeneity, and memory.

Heterogeneity is the ability to respond specifically to a variety of substances.

Memory (anamnestic response) is the ability to recognize and respond to a substance previously encountered.

Innate immunity/resistance—genetically predetermined immunity or resistance that an individual is born with, including **species resistance**.

Acquired immunity is specific immunity developed during an individual's lifetime.

Actively acquired immunity involves the production of antibodies or specialized lymphocytes in response to exposure to an antigen; it is usually long lasting.

Passively acquired immunity—antibodies produced by another source are transferred to an individual to confer immunity; they are generally not long lasting.

Naturally acquired active immunity is a result of an infection.

Artificially acquired active immunity is a result of vaccination.

Naturally acquired passive immunity involves transfer of antibodies from mother to fetus (via the placenta) or from mother to newborn (via the colostrum).

Artificially acquired passive immunity involves acquisition of antibodies by injection.

An **antigen** is a chemical substance (usually foreign) that elicits a specific immune response. It may be a protein, glycoprotein, lipoprotein, nucleoprotein, or large polysaccharide.

An **antibody (immunoglobulin)** is a protein produced by B lymphocytes in response to an antigen. Antibodies bind to antigenic determinant sites or epitopes on the antigen. There are five different immunoglobulin (Ig) classes: IgG, IgM, IgA, IgD, and IgE.

IgG antibodies provide naturally acquired passive immunity; they enhance phagocytosis, neutralize toxins and viruses, participate in complement fixation, and protect both fetus and newborn.

IgM antibodies are the first antibodies produced in response to an infection; they are involved in agglutination and complement fixation.

IgA antibodies protect mucosal surfaces.

IgD antibodies appear to be involved in initiation of the immune response.

IgE antibodies are involved in allergic reactions and possibly in responding to protozoal infections.

There are two components of the immune system: **humoral immunity** and **cell-mediated immunity.**

Humoral immunity is involved in defense against toxins, bacteria, and viruses in *extracellular body fluids* such as plasma and lymph.

Cellular immunity (cell-mediated immunity) is involved in the body's response to multicellular parasites, transplanted tissues, cancer cells, and intracellular viruses. T cells do have receptors for antigens, but they do not make antibodies.

Lymphocytes differentiate into either **B cells** (which are involved in humoral immunity) or **T cells** (which are involved in the cell-mediated response).

B-cells are a type of lymphocyte derived from bone marrow stem cells. They later mature to synthesize and secrete antibodies, which are involved in humoral immunity.

T cells are the lymphocytes of the cell-mediated branch of the acquired immune response. T cells mature in the thymus but derive from the progenitor lymphocytes located in the bone marrow. Once T cells have become activated, they differentiate into specialized T cells, each responsible for a different immune response.

Helper T cells are the control cells of the cell-mediated response. These cells contain **CD4 receptors** on the cell surfaces. Their function is to secrete chemical messengers, which regulate the response of other cells in the immune response. Helper T cells are required to activate cytotoxic T cells. B cells must be activated by T helper cells in order to produce antibodies.

Cytotoxic T cells destroy cells that display abnormal cell surface proteins. These cells contain **CD8 receptors** on the cell surfaces. Cytotoxic T cells destroy cells that have been infected with viruses or intracellular bacteria. These cytotoxic T cells also destroy cancer cells. T cells may also be involved in the defense against certain protozoan and helminthic infections.

Delayed hypersensitivity T cells are involved in allergic reactions and in rejection of transplanted tissue. These may also be involved in the defense against cancer.

Suppressor T cells are involved in turning the immune response off. Suppressor T cells are CD8 positive but may not be cytotoxic T cells.

Natural killer cells (NK cells) are like T cells in that they are capable of killing other cells. However, unlike T cells, these NK cells are not produced in response to a specific antigen.

Cytokines or **lymphokines** are chemical messengers produced by the cells of the immune system that regulate the immune response. Lymphokines are chemical messengers produced by lymphocytes. The term cytokines refers to all chemical messengers produced by cells. **Interleukins** are chemical messengers that act between leukocytes.

Vaccines and **toxoids** (inactivated toxins) are used to confer active immunization.

Vaccines can be made from live attenuated (weakened) organisms, parts of organisms (subunit vaccines), or dead organisms. **Subunit vaccines** are generally safer than either attenuated organisms or whole killed cells. **Recombinant vaccines**, in which the antigen genes of pathogens are inserted into the DNA of a nonpathogen, are very safe.

10.7.3 Immunological Disorders

Immunological disorders include inappropriate responses (hypersensitivity) and inadequate responses (immunodeficiency).

Hypersensitivity (allergy) is an inappropriate response to an antigen that leads to tissue damage rather than immunity. There are four classes of hypersensitivity: the first three (types I, II, and III) are based on humoral immunity, and the reactions occur within seconds or minutes (type I) or hours (types II and III); type IV, a cell-mediated response, is a delayed reaction, usually occurring within 24–48 hours from the time of exposure.

Type I hypersensitivity (anaphylaxis)—a hypersensitivity reaction involving the production of IgE antibodies that bind to basophils and mast cells; it is characterized by the release of histamine, leukotrienes, and prostaglandins, which cause the characteristic allergic reaction.

Asthma, hives, and hay fever are **localized anaphylactic** reactions; **systemic anaphylaxis**, which may develop rapidly upon antigen exposure, may result in circulatory collapse and death.

Allergies are treated by **hyposensitization (desensitization)**, the repeated injection of increasing concentrations of minute amounts of the allergin. **Antihistamines** are used to treat symptoms.

92

Type II hypersensitivity (cytotoxic reactions) are the result of mismatched cellular antigens; IgG or IgM antibodies and complement are involved in the destruction of the foreign cells through lysis or phagocytosis.

Transfusion reactions involve mismatches in the ABO blood group or Rh factor and cause cytotoxic reactions.

Hemolytic disease of a newborn occurs when a woman lacking the Rh antigen (said to be Rh-negative) produces anti-Rh antibodies against an Rh-positive fetus.

Type III hypersensitivity (immune complex diseases)—small complexes of IgG antibodies and soluble antigen are deposited in the basement membranes of cells, activating complement. **Complement fixation** then causes inflammation. An **Arthus reaction** is a localized response of this type.

Rheumatoid arthritis, systemic lupus erythematosus, glomerulonephritis, and serum sickness are immune complex disorders.

Type IV hypersensitivity (cell-mediated hypersensitivity) reactions involve T cells, lymphokines, and macrophages, and result in tissue damage.

Contact dermatitis (e.g., from exposure to poison ivy) and tuberculin skin tests are examples of these types of reactions.

Autoimmune disorders involve the development of hypersensitivity to self, as if the self were a foreign substance. They may result in tissue damage from type II, III, or IV reactions. Rheumatoid arthritis and systemic lupus erythematosus are autoimmune diseases.

Histocompatibility antigens occur on the surface membranes of all cells. Human leukocyte antigens (HLAs) are often involved in transplant rejection.

Donor and recipient are matched as closely as possible with regard to HLA and ABO blood group antigens to decrease the chance of rejection.

Patients that have already been sensitized may experience acute graft rejection (a type II response). Slower rejections are usually due to cell-mediated reactions.

Immune deficiencies may be inherited or acquired. There are also many diseases that can impair immune response.

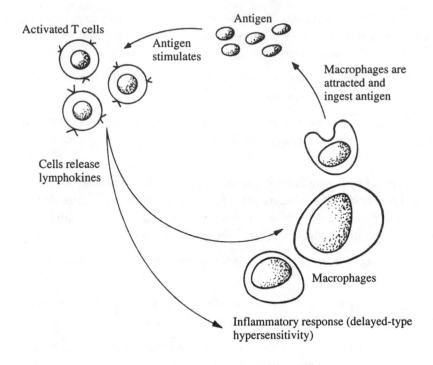

Figure 10.1 Cell-Mediated Immunity

10.7.4 HIV

Human immunodeficiency virus (HIV) is an enveloped retrovirus. An envelope protein is gp120, which attaches to the CD4 cell surface receptor of helper T cells. Once the virus has attached to a CD4 cell, the viral RNA enters the host cell and is transcribed by reverse transcriptase. The resultant DNA molecule is then integrated into the host DNA and begins the production of viral proteins and viral RNAs for repackaging of new virus molecules. Once the virus has reassembled, it is enveloped in the host cell membrane, which contains viral-enveloped proteins, and is once more an infective HIV virus particle.

HIV can be transmitted through infected bodily fluids such as semen, breast milk, and blood. Chemotherapy for HIV infections and treatment of acquired immune deficiency syndrome (AIDS) is directed at reverse transcriptase.

Zidovudine (AZT), ddI, and ddC are nucleotide analogues that inhibit reverse transcriptase activity. Because reverse transcriptase is a specific enzyme to the retrovirus, these nucleotide analogues do not affect significantly the normal replication of host DNA. In addition, the protease is a viral protein vital for the production of functional viral proteins. Protease inhibitors stop the action of the protease and prevent the production of these viral proteins.

Researchers are also working to produce an effective vaccine against the HIV virus. The HIV genome is highly susceptible to mutation. This enables the virus to evade chemotherapy treatments and vaccines by constantly varying the chemical constituency of the viral proteins.

10.8 Microbial Diseases of the Skin and Eyes

Bacterial diseases of the skin include staphylococcal, streptococcal, and pseudomonad infections. Most of these organisms are opportunists, generally part of the normal flora, that gain access through cuts, burns, or surgical incisions. Staph infections can be very difficult to treat; at present, there is only one antibiotic (vancomycin) to which *Staphylococcus aureus* is not resistant. In all likelihood, *S. aureus* will develop resistance to vancomycin at some point as well.

Acne is caused by the bacterium *Propionibacterium acnes*, which metabolizes sebum in hair follicles. The fatty acid end products of this metabolism cause inflammation. The condition is treated with tetracycline and benzoyl peroxide.

Viral diseases of the skin include smallpox, chicken pox, shingles, herpes, measles, rubella, and warts.

Fungal skin diseases include athlete's foot, ringworm, and candidiasis.

Diseases of the eye include conjunctivitis, which is caused by a number of bacteria, and keratitis, which can be caused by a herpes simplex type 1 or *Acanthamoeba*.

The eyes of all newborns are treated with a silver nitrate solution to prevent **neonatal gonorrheal ophthalmia**, which is caused by transmission of *Neisseria gonorrhoeae* from an infected mother to her infant during passage through the birth canal.

10.9   Microbial Diseases of the Respiratory System

Infections of the upper respiratory system can be caused by several bacteria and viruses, often in combination. They include pharyngitis, laryngitis, bronchitis, epiglottitis, and sinusitis.

Bacterial diseases of the upper respiratory system include strep throat (caused by group A beta-hemolytic streptococci), scarlet fever, diphtheria, and otitis media (middle ear infections).

The **common cold** is caused by about 200 different viruses; about half are rhinoviruses. Ear infections and sinus infections may occur as complications.

Bacterial diseases of the lower respiratory system include whooping cough, tuberculosis, and pneumonia.

Tuberculosis is a major, worldwide health problem, and its incidence is increasing in the United States. It is caused by *Mycobacterium tuberculosis*.

Pneumonia is often caused by members of the normal flora. Most infections are due to *Streptococcus pneumoniae, Haemophilus influenzae, Staphylococcus aureus, Legionella pneumophila*, and *Mycoplasma pneumoniae*. *Klebsiella* pneumonia, a rarer form of pneumonia, has an 85% mortality rate.

Viral infections cause influenza and pneumonia as well. The influenza virus exhibits antigenic variation.

Fungal diseases of the lower respiratory system, including histoplasmosis, coccidioidomycosis, and blastomycosis, are treated with amphotericin B.

Pneumocystis carinii infects the lower respiratory system of immunosuppressed or immunocompromised individuals. The taxonomic affiliation (fungus or protozoan) is unclear.

10.10 Microbial Diseases of the Digestive System

Tooth decay (dental caries) and **periodontal disease**—*Streptococcus mutans* is involved in the production of plaque. Bacterial acids destroy tooth enamel, and filamentous bacteria and gram-positive rods invade the underlying dentin and pulp. Gram-negative anaerobes, streptococci, and actinomycetes can cause gingivitis and decay of the underlying cementum, leading to periodontal disease.

Gastrointestinal distress can be caused by pathogens growing in the intestine or from the ingestion of toxins (**bacterial intoxication**). Both infections and intoxications can cause diarrhea, dysentery, or gastroenteritis.

Staphylococcal enterotoxicosis—food poisoning due to ingestion of an enterotoxin found in improperly stored foods.

The exotoxin produced by *Staphylococcus aureus* is not denatured by boiling.

Salmonella gastroenteritis is preventable by heating food to 68°C. It can be caused by many *Salmonella* species. Other bacterial diseases of the lower gastrointestinal tract include typhoid fever (due to *Salmonella typhi* infection), cholera (due to *Vibrio cholerae* exotoxin), *Vibrio parahaemolyticus* gastroenteritis from contaminated mollusks or crustaceans, and *Escherichia coli* gastroenteritis (traveler's diarrhea).

Helicobacter pylori is the cause of **peptic ulcer disease (PUD)**. *H. pylori* binds to the epithelium of the stomach and can grow in the highly acidic environment. This infection causes an immune response and inflammation. In combination with the acid content of the stomach, the inflammation can progress to ulcerated tissue and PUD. The treatment of PUD is now antibiotic treatment in combination with bismuth subsalicylate.

Viral diseases of the digestive tract include mumps and hepatitis.

Fungal diseases of the digestive system include ergot poisoning and aflatoxin poisoning. Mycotoxins (fungal toxins) can affect the blood, nervous system, liver, or kidneys.

There are a number of protozoan diseases of the digestive system, including *Giardia lamblia* infection (giardiasis), amoebic dysentery (amoebiasis), and *Cryptosporidium* infection.

Helminths also cause diseases in the gastrointestinal tract: nematode infestations (pinworms, hookworms, and trichinosis) and tapeworm infestation.

10.11 Microbial Diseases of the Cardiovascular System

Septicemia—growth of microorganisms in the blood—can cause inflamed lymph vessels (**lymphangitis**), septic shock, and decreased blood pressure.

Symptoms are usually the result of endotoxins.

Puerperal sepsis is a uterine infection following childbirth or abortion; it is usually caused by *Streptococcus pyogenes*.

Bacterial endocarditis—infection (usually streptococcal or staphylococcal) of the inner layer of the heart.

Rheumatic fever—a possible complication following streptococcal infection.

Bacteria, such as *Pasteurella multocida*, can be introduced by animal bites and scratches (especially cats, dogs, and rats).

Viral diseases include infectious mononucleosis, yellow fever, and dengue virus.

Protozoans cause toxoplasmosis, malaria, and Chagas' disease.

Schistosomiasis and swimmer's itch are helminthic diseases.

10.12 Microbial Diseases of the Nervous System

Bacterial meningitis can be caused by nearly 50 species of opportunistic bacteria, including *Neisseria meningitidis*, *Haemophilus influenzae*, and *Streptococcus pneumoniae*.

Leprosy, tetanus, and botulism are also caused by bacteria.

Viral diseases include poliomyelitis, rabies, and arthropod-borne encephalitis.

Fungal diseases include *Cryptococcus* meningitis.

Protozoal diseases include *Naegleria* meningoencephalitis and African trypanosomiasis.

10.13 Microbial Diseases of the Genitourinary System

Bacterial diseases of the urinary system include cystitis, glomerulonephritis, and pyelonephritis.

Bacterial diseases of the reproductive system include gonorrhea, nongono-coccal urethritis, syphilis, vaginitis, chancroid, granuloma inguinale, and lymphogranuloma venereum.

Viral diseases of the reproductive system include cytomegalovirus, genital herpes, and genital warts.

Candidiasis, a fungal disease, and trichomoniasis, a protozoal disease, also affect the genitourinary system.

CHAPTER 11

Microbes in the Environment

11.1 Microbes and the Recycling of Nutrients

Microbes, especially bacteria and fungi, play an important role in the **decomposition** of organic matter and the **recycling** of chemical elements.

Bioconversion is the microbial conversion of organic waste materials into alternative fuels.

Bioremediation is the use of bacteria to clean up toxic wastes.

11.1.1 Biogeochemical Cycles

Microbes are essential to the **recycling** of chemical elements such as carbon, nitrogen, phosphorus, sulfur, and oxygen.

They also **solubilize minerals**, such as sulfur, potassium, iron, and others, making them available for plant metabolism.

The carbon cycle—photoautotrophs fix CO_2, providing nutrients for chemoheterotrophs. Chemoheterotrophs release CO_2, which can then be used by the photoautotrophs.

The nitrogen cycle—bacteria are involved in the decomposition of proteins from dead cells, ammonification of the amino acids, and reduction of nitrates to molecular nitrogen (N_2). Nitrogen-fixing bacteria are responsible for converting molecular nitrogen back into ammonium and nitrate, which can then be used by other bacteria and plants in the synthesis of amino acids.

11.1.2 Microbes in the Soil, Water, and Air

Microbes from all taxonomic groups are present in the soil.

Soil contains inorganic material (rocks, minerals, water, and gases) as well as organic matter (humus) and microorganisms.

Microbes from all taxonomic groups are present in both freshwater and marine environments. However, the high osmotic pressure, low nutrient availability, and high pH of the open ocean makes the marine environment unfavorable for many microbes.

Many pathogens are transmitted in drinking water. Bacterial counts are used in assaying water purity.

Sewage treatment—aerobic bacteria are used to decompose organic matter in secondary treatment of sewage waste.

Microbes do not live in the air, but can be transmitted through the air.

11.2   Bioremediation

Bioremediation is the concerted effort by researchers and scientists to increase the activity of those microorganisms that effectively degrade pollution. Certain types of bacteria are able to degrade petroleum but require the addition of nitrogen and phosphorus to encourage bacterial growth. Oxygen is also required for this process, and contaminated soil must be constantly aerated in order to encourage bacterial degradation of petroleum spills.

Bacteria also are able to naturally degrade or chemically process heavy metals, sulfur, nitrogen gas, and polychlorinated biphenyls (PCBs). These bacteria may also be genetically altered to increase their natural ability to degrade these pollutants. This solution to pollution is attractive because it converts a potentially harmful substance to a harmless or useful substance.

Pseudomonads are capable of converting methyl mercury, a highly toxic form of mercury, to mercuric ion and then to elemental mercury, a relatively nontoxic element.

CHAPTER 12

Microbes in Industry

12.1 Microbes in the Food Industry

Alcoholic beverages and vinegar—fermentation by yeasts is responsible for the production of ethanol; *Acetobacter* and *Gluconobacter* oxidize the alcohol in wine to acetic acid (vinegar).

Cheese—lactic acid bacteria are used to curdle cheese and in the production of hard cheeses.

Lactobacilli, streptococci, and yeasts are used in the production of buttermilk, sour cream, and yogurt.

Nondairy fermentation by various microbes is involved in making sauerkraut, pickles, olives, and soy sauce. The fermentation of yeast produces ethanol and CO_2, which makes bread dough rise.

12.2 Industrial Microbiology

Industrial microbiology—use of microbes to manufacture or help manufacture useful products or to dispose of waste.

Microbes can produce acetone, alcohols, glycerol, and organic acids.

Some microbes, e.g., *Thiobacillus ferrooxidans*, can extract mineral ores. Minerals that can be extracted include arsenic, copper, uranium, iron, cobalt, lead, nickel, and zinc.

A large number of enzymes are commercially produced by microorganisms. For example, **alpha amylase** is produced by *Aspergillus niger* or *Aspergillus oryzae*. This enzyme is used as a flour supplement in baking, in the textile industry, and in the pharmaceutical industry as a digestive aid for beans. *Bacillus subtilis* is a major producer of alpha amylase used in brewing. The enzyme **beta amylase** is produced by a variety of microorganisms and is used for the production of maltose syrup. **Invertase** is produced by *Saccharomyces cervisiae* in the production of candy and artificial honey. **Streptokinase** is produced by *Streptococcus* (spp.) as an exotoxin and is used in medicine to lyse embolisms and thrombolisms.

12.3 Microbes and Medicine

Pharmaceutical microbiology—use of microbes to manufacture products used in medicine.

Bacteria produce most of the amino acids used in medicine and food.

Microbes can produce antibiotics, enzymes, vitamins, and hormones.

12.4 Microbes and Recombinant DNA Technology

The ability to genetically engineer cells has paved the way for the production of many new products.

12.4.1 Applications in Medicine

Currently, such important substances as insulin and interferon are produced from genetically engineered microorganisms.

Synthetic genes for the two polypeptides that make up **human insulin** have been inserted into a plasmid vector and transferred into *E. coli* for production and secretion. Mammalian cells are also used to produce insulin.

Cells can be engineered to produce surface proteins of pathogens for use as **subunit vaccines**. Animal viruses can be used to engineer **recombinant vaccines**, e.g., the antigen genes from a pathogenic microorganism can be inserted into the DNA of a nonpathogenic microbe.

The **polymerase chain reaction** is used to enzymatically produce multiple copies of a piece of DNA, and to increase amounts of DNA in samples to detectable levels so that they may be used in gene sequencing and other diagnostic procedures.

DNA probes provide rapid identification of pathogens in food and body tissues.

12.4.2 Applications in Agriculture

Cells from plants with the desired characteristics can be cloned.

The vector most often used for the transfer of plant DNA is the **Ti plasmid** inserted into *Agrobacterium*. *Agrobacterium* is a bacterium that naturally transforms plant cells. Thus, *Agrobacterium* readily transfers genes to plants and, as such, is a very useful tool in genetic engineering.

E. coli is used to produce bovine growth hormone.

12.4.3 Safety Issues

There are strict safety standards for the development and use of genetically engineered microorganisms.

One technique for decreasing the probability that a genetically engineered microbe will survive outside the lab or beyond a certain time limit is to insert so-called **suicide genes** into them along with the gene of interest.

12.4.4 The Future of Genetic Engineering

Genetic engineering should continue to provide us with new diagnostic tools and treatments for disease.